DERMATOLOGY - LABORATORY AND CLINICAL RESEARCH

INFLAMMATORY MARKERS, ONCOGENES, TUMOR SUPPRESSOR CELL CYCLE REGULATORS IN SKIN GROWTHS, PRE-SKIN TUMORS AND SKIN TUMORS

DERMATOLOGY - LABORATORY AND CLINICAL RESEARCH

Additional books in this series can be found on Nova's website under the Series tab.

Additional e-books in this series can be found on Nova's website under the e-book tab.

DERMATOLOGY - LABORATORY AND CLINICAL RESEARCH

INFLAMMATORY MARKERS, ONCOGENES, TUMOR SUPPRESSOR CELL CYCLE REGULATORS IN SKIN GROWTHS, PRE-SKIN TUMORS AND SKIN TUMORS

ANA MARIA ABREU VELEZ
EDITOR

NOVA BIOMEDICAL
New York

Additional color graphics may be available in the e-book version of this book.

Library of Congress Cataloging-in-Publication Data

ISBN: 978-1-63484-303-4
Library of Congress Control Number: 2015957364

Published by Nova Science Publishers, Inc. † New York

CONTENTS

PREFACE

Inflammatory markers, oncogenes, tumor suppressor genes and cell cycle regulators in skin growths represent a series of reports and reviews on skin cancers and precancers, their host immune responses and correlations with medical literature data.

We were able to clearly identify an immune response in multiple skin cancers, as well as in cutaneous pre-cancerous conditions. In poorly differentiated tumor areas, some classic immunohistochemical stains did not stain as frequently described in the literature.

Other important phenomena we observed are that many cell cycle regulators, cell cycle checkpoints, oncogenes and tumor suppressor gene markers were not only positive inside the tumors, but also in cells around the tumor. Portions of adjacent skin appendices and in supposedly normal adjacent epidermal and dermal tissue also showed signs of these components. These common findings raised questions concerning marginal definition of cutaneous surgery; that is, many of the immunologic findings could not be correlated on classical hematoxylin and eosin reviews.

We also noted that many immunologic cells around skin cancers and/or pre-cancers showed high rates of division defined via markers such as Ki-67; our findings utilizing double color immunohistochemistry also showed that these immune cells are possibly actively duplicating as effector cells. Ki-67 has been cited as a superb proliferation marker in melanoma, but additional review of its utility is warranted given our results.

Finally, we also found double staining immunohistochemistry to be of excellent value in detecting melanoma cells metastasizing in blood vessels, lymphatics and/or nerves.

Ana Maria Abreu Velez, MD, PhD
Georgia Dermatopathology Associates
1534 North Decatur Road., NE, Suite 206
Atlanta, Georgia 30307-1000 US
Telephone: (404) 371-0077
Toll Free: (877) 371-0027
Fax: (404) 371-1900
E-mail: abreuvelez@yahoo.com

In: Inflammatory Markers, Oncogenes … ISBN: 978-1-63484-303-4
Editor: Ana Maria Abreu Velez

Chapter 1

INFLAMMATORY MARKERS, ONCOGENES, AND TUMOR SUPPRESSOR CELL CYCLE REGULATORS IN BENIGN, PREMALIGNANT AND MALIGNANT SKIN LESIONS

Ana Maria Abreu-Vélez[1,*], MD, PhD, Juliana Calle-Isaza[2], MD, Yulieth Alexandra Upegui-Zapata[3], MSc, Daniel Alberto Vásquez-Hincapié[3], MD, Eduardo Upegui-Quiceño, EdS, LPC, Natalia Regina Mesa-Herrera[4], PhD, Carlos Andrés Valencia-Yepes[5], MSc, Jorge Enrique Velasquez-Velez[6], MD and Michael S. Howard[1], MD

[1]Georgia Dermatopathology Associates, Atlanta, Georgia, US
[2]Clinica Medellin el Poblado, Colombia, South America
[3]PECET, University of Antioquia,Medellín, Colombia, South America
[4]University of Antioquia, Medellín, Colombia, South America
[5]Gobernacion de Antioquia, Medellín, Colombia, South America
[6]Clinica Ces, Colombia, South America

* Corresponding author: Ana Maria Abreu Velez, MD, PhD, Georgia Dermatopathology Associates, 1534 North Decatur Road., NE; Suite 206; Atlanta, Georgia 30307-1000 US. E-mail: abreuvelez@yahoo.com, tel.: (404) 371-0077, toll free: (877) 371-0027, fax: (404) 371-1900.

ABSTRACT

There is an increasing interest in understanding the roles of the immune system, cell cycle regulations, tumor suppressor genes and oncogenes in the development and progression of pre- skin cancers and skin cancers. The significance of these in human skin cancer has been documented based primarily upon the augmented incidence of skin cancers in organ transplant recipients, patients with some genodermatosis that predispose them to skin cancer and the increase of ultraviolet (UV) radiation-mediated immunomodulation. In this review, we incorporate multiple lines of evidence emphasizing the role that immune system cell cycle regulators have on pre-skin cancers and skin cancers. These entities include actinic keratosis, actinic cheilitis, leukoplakia, keratoacanthoma, Bowen's disease, dysplastic nevus, squamous cell carcinoma, basal cell carcinoma, Merkel cell carcinoma, neurofibroma, perineuromas, cutaneous hyperneury, schwannoma, extramammary Paget's disease, dermatofibrosarcoma protuberans, pleomorphic dermal sarcoma and others. The interaction between the immune systems and oncogenes, tumor suppressor molecules, and altered cell cycle regulators are consider in this review, as well as immunomodulatory therapies.

Keywords: oncogenes, tumor suppressor and cell cycle regulators in skin growths, pre-skin and skin tumors, skin cancer, melanoma, actinic keratoses, squamous cell carcinoma, basal cell carcinoma, sarcoma, merkel cell carcinoma, cutaneous lymphoma, oncogenes, tumor suppressor genes, immune response

ABBREVIATIONS AND ACRONYMS

AK	Actinic keratoses
SCC	squamous cell carcinoma
BCC	basal cell carcinoma
NBCCS	nevoid basal cell carcinoma syndrome
TSGs	tumor suppressor genes
UV	ultraviolet
PDT	photodynamic therapy
IHC	immunohistochemistry
AD	autosomal dominant
5-FU	5-fluorouracil
MMS	Mohs micrographic surgery

PCNA	hematoxylin and eosin (H and E) staining, proliferating cell nuclear antigen
BCL-2	B-cell lymphoma 2 gene
MART-1	melanoma antigen recognized by T-cells 1 staining
TCA	trichloroacetic acid
FM	familial melanoma
HMB-45	human melanoma black-45
Mel-5	melanoma 5
MART-1	melanoma antigen recognized by T-cells 1
Dox	doxorubicin
CpG	CpGoligodeoxynucleotides
HGNC, Hugo	Hugo Gene Nomenclature Conference Committee
CDKN2A	cyclin-dependent kinase inhibitor 2A
BRAF	v-raf murine sarcoma viral oncogene homolog B1
SOX10	Sry-related HMg-Box gene 10

Pre-Cancers

Certain potentially precancerous growths, or pre-cancers, most of them resulting from cumulative sun damage, can be associated with later development of cancer lesions. One of them is the actinic, or solar keratosis (AK). These rough, scaly, slightly raised growths, ranging in color from brown to red and from about 1 mm to 1 inch in diameter, are found on sun-exposed areas of the body, most often in older people. They may represent the first step to squamous cell carcinoma (SCC), and some experts consider them the earliest form of SCC. From two to ten percent of untreated AKs advance to SCC, sometimes within two years, according to different studies. Indeed, 40 to 60 percent of squamous cell carcinomas begin as untreated AKs.The longer AKs exist untreated and the older these lesions are, the greater the chance that one may develop into an invasive SCC. AKs are often palpable before becoming visible, and can be felt by running your fingers over sun-exposed areas; this can provide an early sign of their presentation. Actinic cheilitis is another form of pre-cancer; this form of AK occurs most often on the lower lip, causing it to become dry, cracked, scaly and pale or white. To make things worse, the patients tend to lick them, often increasing the dryness. Why the lower lip? Because the lower lip receives more sun exposure than the upper lip. If not treated promptly, actinic cheilitis can lead to SCC. If your lips are frequently chapped or burning, you may have actinic cheilitis. Leukoplakia is another pre-cancerous lesion, arising on the mucous membranes; these white patches on the tongue, gums, cheeks, or elsewhere inside the mouth have the potential to develop into SCC. They may be caused by sources of chronic irritation, such as habitual alcohol consumption or tobacco use, or rough edges on teeth or dentures. They may also be caused by a long-time biting habit.

Actinic Keratoses (AK)

AKs are considered a worldwide problem with increasing incidence, especially for the rise in senior population and chronic sun exposure. They clinically present as rough or scaly plaques and are histologically characterized by a proliferation of atypical keratinocytes limited to the lower epidermis [1-8] (Figure 1). AKs are frequently seen on sun-exposed areas e.g., balding scalp, face, lateral neck, and distal upper or lower extremities. AKs are considered to be an early step in the transformation from normal skin to SCC.

These lesions develop on a background of field cancerization, in which chronically ultraviolet (UV) damaged areas accrue molecular changes, but persist "clinically normal" for lengthy periods [1-8].

Epidemiology, Risk Factors and Increased Risk of Disease Progression in AKs

In the United States, AKs are extremely common, especially in individuals with fair skin. These individuals are most likely to develop AKs, and considerable data on the epidemiology and risk factors for AK are derived from studies in Australia, northern Europe, and the United States. Factors such as the extent of exposure to UV and certain phenotypic features have been associated with a risk of developing these lesions [1-8]. The presence of certain clinical features in AKs, including large size, ulceration, or bleeding, suggests progression to SCC.

The risk is also increased by extensive solar or other UV damage, advanced age, and immune suppression [1-8]. Please see Table 1 for suggestions for people susceptible to develop pre-skin or skin cancers.

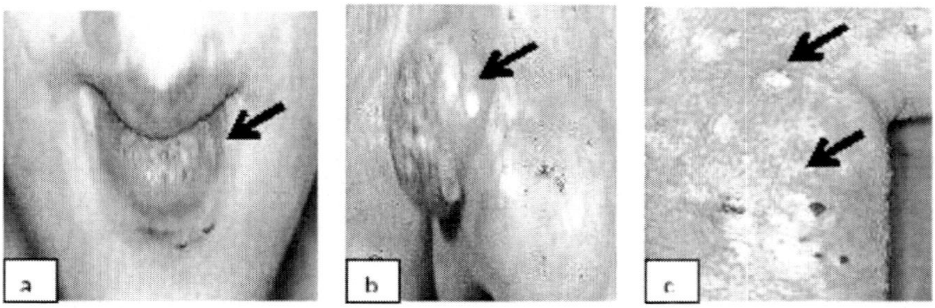

Figure 1. a, shows a clinical example of lower lip cheilitis, b of basal cell carcinoma in the nose c of actinic keratosis and squamous cell carcinoma (black arrows).

Table 1. Suggestions for people susceptible to develop pre-skin and or skin cancers

Try to find the shade, especially between 10 AM and 4 PM if you go to the beach, walks, vacation, and gardening and or of you have to workevery day under the exposure of sun or UV.
Evade suntan and or sun exposure to the point of burning your skin. It is believe that this can increase the risk of development of skin cancer.
Sidestepof recurrent tanning even if "is hot" and try to avoid the use UV tanning beds.
Cover up with clothing especially with cotton, and white and or light colors that, including a broad overflowed hat and UV-blocking sunglasses.
Use a broad spectrum (UVA/UVB) sunscreen with an SPF of 15 or higher every day. For extended outdoor activity, use a water-resistant, broad spectrum (UVA/UVB) sunscreen with an SPF of 30 or higher. If you are hiking or doing any outdoor activity and or work search for an area that have shadows and try to do the work under the shadows
Apply 1 ounce (2 tablespoons) of sunscreen to your entire body 30 minutes before going outside. Reapply every two hours or after swimming or excessive sweating.
If you have a newborns with icteric, put on the sun avoiding the exposure between 10 am to 4pm and only put on the sun for 5 minutes each side of the body covering the baby eyes with some piece of cloth. Sunscreens should be used on babies over the age of six months.
Inspect your skin head-to-toe in a regular base and you or your family has history of skin cancer visit the dermatologist every six months. You can self-examine for moles o skin changes monthly.
Eat carrots or food rich in carotenes such papaya is you have to be expose to sun.

Treatment Modalities for AK

Management of the specific actinic damaged skin is the best treatment, although recent developments have focused on the management of the whole actinically damaged field (Table 1). In this regard, several topical drugs have been approved, differing in efficacy, side effects, application and cost. Research continuously aims to develop the "ideal" treatment which combines high clearance rates with few side effects, short treatment duration and low costs. Multiple treatments are available, some have a long track history of success such as topical 5-fluorouracil (5-FU) at 5% (Fluoroplex®, Efudex®, Carac®) cream, that acts by directly attacking the precancerous cells. The cream is applied once to twice daily for 2 to 4 weeks [9-14]. Usually it is applied at night, since it can be irritating. It is also common to send a topical mild to medium strength corticosteroid cream, to be applied a few minutes later after the 5-FU. Some patients cannot tolerate the "burning" of the skin and the pain, and it is wise to allow them to rest one to three days after applying the cream and restart later when their tolerance is better [9-14]. Treatment leaves the affected area temporarily reddened and raw, and will cause some discomfort. The authors believe this is the best treatment available for AK because the 5-FU only acts on the cells that have abnormal growth and altered cell cycle division [9-14].

Cryosurgery

One of the most common treatments done for AKs; lesions are frozen off, through the application of liquid nitrogen [9-14]. This is done with a special spray device or cotton-tipped applicator; however, the applicator does not reach the optimal freezing point. Cryosurgery does not require anesthesia and produces no bleeding, but causes discomfort in the patient. The longer the lesion is frozen, the better the chance it will never come back [9-14]. Longer freezing can result in hypopigmented areas. The authors have not experienced the qualityresults with this technique, relative to 5-FU.

Electrocoagulation with Hyfrecator, and Curettage

Represents another treatment for AK. The physician can administer local anesthesia, and then electrocoagulate the AK using a hyfrecator. The hyfrecator is a low-powered medical apparatus used in electrosurgery, on conscious patients, usually in an office setting [9-14]. It is used to destroy tissue directly, and to stop bleeding during minor surgery while scraping the lesions.

If electrocoagulation is not done, it is possible to take a biopsy specimen foe hematoxylin and eosin (H and E) review. The bleeding is controlled by cautery, i.e., via application of an acid or heat produced by an electric device [9-14].

Shave Removal

Utilizes a scalpel and/or skin biopsy device to shave the AK, and obtain a specimen for testing. The base of the lesion is destroyed, and the bleeding is stopped by cauterization [9-14]. Thebiopsy specimen is submitted for H and E review.

Chemical Peels

The use of acids such the Jessner's solution and/or trichloroacetic acid (TCA), applied to the AK. Jessner's solution is a combination of superficial peeling agents, i.e., salicylic acid, resorcinol and lactic acid. It goes a little deeper than a glycolic acid peel [9-14]. The peel goes through the epidermis, to the junction of the epidermis and dermis. It is also used as a first step in deeper peels, such as a 35% TCA with Jessner's. The top layers of the skin peel off, and are usually replaced within seven days by the growth of new skin. Redness and soreness usually disappear after a few days [9-14].

Topical Imiquimod Cream

Topical cream is effective in treating AKs, particularly when lesions are abundant. One of the latest medications, imiquimod cream, works by stimulating the body's immune system to identify these precancerous lesions and destroy them [9-14]. This is used twice weekly for 6-12 weeks over the affected areas (Table 1).

Solaraze® Gel

Solaraze gel is a non-steroidal medication that also works fairly well on AK's. Treatment with Solaraze is twice daily for ninety days [9-14].

Photodynamic Therapy (PDT)

PDT, sometimes called photochemotherapy, is a form of phototherapy using nontoxic light-sensitive compounds that are exposed selectively to light; upon exposure they become toxic to targeted malignant and other diseased cells (phototoxicity) [9-14].

PDT has three steps. 1) A light-sensitizing liquid, cream, or intravenous drug (photosensitizer) is applied or administered.

In some cases, a photosensitizing molecule that is already in the body can be utilized. 2) There is an incubation period of minutes to days. 3) The target tissue is then exposed to a specific wavelength of light, that activates the photosensitizing medication.

In dermatology, PDT with the photosensitizer LevulanKerastick® (20% delta-aminolevulinic acid HCl) is used for the treatment of AKs [9-14]. The initial FDA approval was specifically for the treatment of AK of the face and scalp; certain other types of cancer cells can be eliminated this way. Current PDT therapy involves a diversity of incubation times for different light-sensitizing drugs, and a variety of light sources depending on the target tissue [9-14].

The therapeutic advantage of PDT is selective tissue destruction. The main limitation of PDT techniques is the depth of penetration of the light, and thus the inability to target cells more than 1/3 of an inch (approximately 1 cm) below the skin surface. Therefore, tumors or atypical growths must be close to the surface of the skin for PDT to work [9-14]. Wide local excision or surgical removalis also a classical treatment for AK [9-14].

Mohs Micrographic Surgery (MMS)

Has become widely utilized for surgical excision of non-melanoma skin cancers, for efficiency and maximal preservation of normal tissue. MMS entails processing specimens in horizontal frozen sections with immediate examination under a light microscope. This technique offers the examination of lateral and deep margins in the same plane [15-20].

Success with MMS depends on accurate mapping of the tumor, correct interpretation of the histopathological sections, and appreciation of aggressive tumor characteristics.

Because H and E staining may present difficulties in the interpretation of frozen sections, rapid immunohistochemistry (IHC) may be warranted [15-20]. MMS is invaluable in the treatment of aggressive and high-risk cutaneous neoplasms, in order to achieve tumor-free margins. IHC as an adjunct to MMS facilitates identification of otherwise hard-to-detect neoplastic cells, thereby increasing the procedure's sensitivity.

By harnessing the appropriate application of IHC to specific tumors, the MMS surgeon is better equipped to maximize tissue sparing and minimize tumor recurrence. IHC offers a broad arena for continued research and further advances in MMS techniques [15-20].

Immune Response in Actinic Keratosis

The association between AKs and the immune system has been previouslyinvestigated, but is poorly understood. In this book, we report a case of an inflamed AK and the associated immune response.

It is known that that seniors and immunocompromised patients are at increased risk of developing AKs [21, 22]. The risk is mainly enhanced at sites that receive high levels of ultraviolet exposure from the sun, which is thought to be a driver of DNA mutations in the skin.

The immune system appears to play a key role in preventing these mutations from progressing to malignant disease, and/or local expansion. The mechanisms involved in this immune-based process remain elusive [21, 22].

Basal Cell Carcinoma (BCC)

BCCs are the most common skin cancer and are abnormal, uncontrolled growths or lesions that arise from the skin's basaloid keratinocytes, which are present in the deepest layer of the epidermis. BCCs often look like pearly micropapules, sometime with telangiectasias; they may also present as ulcers, red-pink patches, shiny bumps, or scars.

BCCs are usually caused by a combination of cumulative and intense, occasional sun exposure (Figure 1) [23-28]. BCC rarely metastasizes beyond the original tumor site. Multiple cases of BCC demonstrate an overactive Sonic Hedgehog signaling pathway (tumor suppressor genes), (TSG) [23-28]. The nevoid basal cell carcinoma syndrome (NBCCS) is an autosomal dominant disorder that manifests as multiple BCCs, pits of the palms and soles, jaw keratocysts, various other tumors, and developmental abnormalities; the candidate gene has been identified at Chromosome 9q22.3 [23-28]. Further, loss of heterozygosity has been demonstrated in the same region in several sporadic BCCs [23-28].

Now termedPTCH, the gene encodes a receptor for the Sonic Hedgehog (SHH) pathway, a pathway important for patterning and growth during vertebrate development [23-28].

The Clinical Diagnosis of BCC

The clinical diagnosis of BCC is not difficult for a trained dermatologist and others medical and paramedical people. The Dermatoscopy can help in the diagnosis [29].

The more common findings in the dermatoscopy (a magnifying device that emits polarized light) shows arborizing telangiectasias, leaf-like areas, foci of microulceration, multiple blue/gray globules, and large blue/gray ovoid nests [29]. Pigmented BCCs can be a diagnostic challenge because they can demonstrate dermatoscopic features suggestive of melanocytic lesions, such as multiple brown-to-black dots/globules, blue/white veil-like structures, and some arborizing vessels [29]. A biopsy is absolutely a must, to confirm the BCC and determine the treatment. Various biopsy techniques may be used, including excisional, incisional, shave, and punch biopsies. Punch and shave biopsies have been shown to have similar diagnostic accuracy and shave biopsies are so superficial, that are the not encourage to be done at all since theydo not show the sides or the deep of the lesion [30-32]. Some histological subtypes of BCC are consider to be most aggressive such as single or mixed histology tumors containing morpheaform, infiltrative, micronodular, or basosquamous components. The immunohistochemistry stains using epithelial antigen, clone (Ber-EP4) is the best for the diagnosis of BCC, but in some undifferentiated cases in our laboratory had shown to be positive such ProliferatingCell Nuclear Antigen (PCNA) and B-cell lymphoma 2 gene (BCL-2) [30-33]. Only in exceedingly rare cases can it spread to other parts of the body and become life-threatening like in the middle line of the face and or in areas of embryological pledges. However the lesions can be disfiguring if not treated promptly [23, 30].

Risk Factors for Developing BCC

Previous history of BCC, familial history of BCC, chronic exposure to sun (including sunburn) and transplants. Anyone with a history of sun exposure can develop BCC. However, people who are at highest risk have fair skin, blond or red hair, and blue, green, or grey eyes. The most common areas of developing BCC are those sun-exposed including the face, nose, ears, neck, scalp, shoulders, and back. On rare occasions, however, tumors develop on unexposed areas. In a few cases, contact with arsenic, exposure to radiation, open sores that resist healing, chronic inflammatory skin conditions, and complications of burns, scars, infections, vaccinations, or even tattoos are contributing factors. It is not possible to pinpoint a precise, single cause for a specific tumor, especially one found on a sun-protected area of the body or in an extremely young individual [23, 30]. The disease is rarely seen in children, but occasionally a teenager is affected. Dermatologists report that more and more people in their twenties and thirties are being treated for this skin cancer. Men with BCC have outnumbered women with the disease.

Risk of Recurrence

People who have had one BCC are at risk for developing others over the years, either in the same area or elsewhere on the body. Therefore, regular visits to a dermatologist should be routine [23, 30]. BCCs on the scalp and nose are especially troublesome, with recurrences typically taking place within the first two years following surgery.

Prevention

While BCCs and other skin cancers are almost always curable when detected and treated early, it is best to prevent them in the first place. Make these sun safety habits part of your daily health care routine: seek the shade, especially between 10 AM and 4 PM, do not burn, avoid tanning and never use UV tanning beds. Cover up with clothing, including a broad-brimmed hat and UV-blocking sunglasses. Use a broad spectrum (UVA/UVB) sunscreen with an SPF of 15 or higher every day. For extended outdoor activity, use a water-resistant, broad spectrum (UVA/UVB) sunscreen with an SPF of 30 or higher. Apply 1 ounce (2 tablespoons) of sunscreen to your entire body 30 minutes before going outside. Reapply every two hours or after swimming or excessive sweating [23, 30]. Keep newborns out of the sun. Sunscreens should be used on babies over the age of six months. Examine your skin head-to-toe every month. See your doctor every year for a professional skin exam [23-30]. If the doctor found a possible BCC, the diagnosis of BCC need to be confirmed with a biopsy. In this procedure, the skin is first numbed with local anesthesia. A sample of the tissue is then removed and sent to be examined under a microscope in the laboratory to seek a definitive diagnosis. For more extensive review on histological types, clinical variants please see reference 23. If tumor cells are present, treatment is required.

Fortunately, there are several effective methods for eliminating BCC. The choice of treatment is based on the type, size, location, and depth of penetration of the tumor, the patient's age and general health, and the likely outcome to his or her appearance.

Treatment can almost always be performed on an outpatient basis in the physician's office or at a clinic. With the various surgical techniques, a local anesthetic is commonly used. Pain or discomfort during the procedure is minimal, and pain afterwards is rare [23-30].

TREATMENTS

Curettage and Electrodesiccation

This technique is usually reserved for small lesions. The growth is scraped off with a curette, an instrument with a sharp, ring-shaped tip), then the tumor site is desiccated (burned) with an electrocautery needle. The procedure has cure rates generally above 95 percent. In some areas of the body, it is repeated a few times to help assure that all cancer cells are eliminated. Local anesthesia is required. The technique may not be as useful for aggressive BCCs, those in high-risk sites, or sites that would be left with cosmetically undesirable results. Typically, a round, whitish scar is left at the surgery site [34].

Mohs Micrographic Surgery

Please see as described above for AK [34]. In recent years, however, efforts to improve and refine the Mohs surgeon's ability to identify melanoma cells have resulted in the development of special stains that highlight these cells. IHC special stains that preferentially stick to pigment cells (melanocytes), where melanoma occurs, making them much easier to see with the microscope. For example, staining excised frozen tissue sections with MART-1 effectively labels/locates the melanocytes, helping to home in on melanomas (Table 3). The MART-1-stained sections are processed and evaluated for the presence of tumor in the margins; certain signs such as nests of atypical melanocytes show that the margins are positive for melanoma and that further surgery must be done. If none of these signs are present, the surgery is concluded. Thanks to such advances, more surgeons are now using the Mohs procedure with certain melanomas.

Excisional Surgery

Using a scalpel, the physician removes the entire growth along with a surrounding border of apparently normal skin as a safety margin. The skin around the surgical site is closed with stitches, and the tissue specimen is sent to the laboratory to verify that all cancerous cells have been removed [35]. It is important that large lesions be removed by a plastic surgeon because it is often needed to use free-flap reconstruction on the defects, and in some cases skin transplant from other parts of the body to cover the area. Cure rates are generally above 95 percent in most body areasand the author prefers this method over curettage and electrodesiccation. A repeat excision may be necessary on a subsequent occasion if evidence of skin cancer is found in the specimen.

Radiation

X-ray beams are directed through the skin at the tumor. Total destruction usually requires several treatments over a few weeks, or sometimes daily for one month. This is ideal for tumors hard to manage surgically and for elderly patients or others in poor health. Cure rates are around 90 percent [34]. Although radiation limits damage to adjacent tissue, it can involve long-term cosmetic problems and radiation risks.

Cryosurgery

Tumor tissue is destroyed by freezing. Liquid nitrogen is applied to the growth with a cotton-tipped applicator or spray device, freezing it without requiring any cutting or anesthesia (though a local anesthetic can be used, since the technique often involves a modest amount of pain) [34]. The experience of the author using cryosurgery is effective for patients with bleeding disorders or intolerance to anesthesia but had higher recurrences.

Photodynamic Therapy (PDT)

PDT is FDA-approved for the treatment of superficial or nodular BCC, with cure rates ranging from 70 to 90 percent. A light-sensitizing agent such, topical 5-aminolevulinic acid (5-ALA), is applied to the lesion in the physician's office [36, 37]. Subsequently, the medicated area is activated by a blue light which theoretically, this will selectively destroys BCCs while causing minimal damage to surrounding normal tissue [36, 37]. However, no larger studies have been published in regards to the damage or not of the surrounding tissue around the BCC. Some redness, pain, and swelling can result. Patients should be advised to avoid sunlight for at least 48 hours, or UV exposure may activate the medication, causing sunburns [36, 37].

Laser Surgery

Some lasers vaporize the skin's top layer to destroy lesions. Others (non-ablative lasers) have been shown to be of use in some cases to treat small, superficial BCC successfully [33-37]. Laser treatments have recurrence rates similar to those of PDT.

Topical Medications

These creams, gels, or solutions are used to treat limited, specific BCC and includes.

Imiquimod

This is FDA-approved only for superficial BCCs, with cure rates generally between 80 and 90 percent. The cream is rubbed gently into the tumor five times a week for up to six weeks or longer [38]. This drugs works by stimulating the immune system, it causes the body to produce interferon, which attacks cancer (Table 2).

5-Fluorouracil (5-FU)

It is a chemotherapy drug approved to treat internal cancers, but it's also useful for AK, and also has been FDA-approved for superficial BCCs, with similar cure rates to imiquimod. The liquid or cream is gently rubbed into the tumor twice a day for three to six weeks [38]. Side effects are variable, and some patients do not experience any discomfort, but redness, irritation, and inflammation usually occur.

Notes

It is important to note that (unlike Mohs surgery and excisional surgery), curettage and electrodesiccation, radiation, cryosurgery, and topical medications all have one significant drawback in common – since no tissue is examined under the microscope, there is no way to determine how completely the tumor was removed.

For these reasons it is important before the use of any of these treatments, first take a skin biopsy to determine the type of BCC and the aggressiveness of the tumor.

Table 2. Topical and systemic immune therapy for skin cancers

Lesions	Topical immune response modifiers	Mechanism of action
AK, superficial BCC and warts. Some success in some cases of squamous cell carcinoma in situ, melanoma and extramammary Paget's disease.	Imiquimod and resiquimod[1].	The stimulation of innate and cell-mediated immune responses through Toll-like receptor-mediated induction of cytokines.
BCC	Vismodegib	Represents the first Hedgehog signaling pathway targeting agent to gain US FDA approval.
Melanoma and none melanoma skin cancer.	TLR7 agonist[2].	Localized TLR7/8 activation.
Melanoma.	Nivolumab[3].	Monoclonal antibody against programmed death receptor-1, an immune checkpoint inhibitor which negatively regulates T-cell proliferation and activation.
Melanona (metastatic)	Dacarbazine[4].	Dacarbazine is a member of the class of alkylating agents, which destroy cancer cells by adding an alkyl group (C_nH_{2n+1}) to its DNA.
Melanoma (metastatic).	Pembrolizumab[5].	Anti-PD1 antibodies. (Block the interaction between the programmed cell death (PD)-1 protein and one of its ligands, PD-L1.
Melanoma (metastatic).	Ipilimumab[5].	Anti-CTLA-4 antibody.
Melanoma (metastatic).	Peginterferon-alfa-2b[5].	Anti-CTLA-4 antibody.
Melanoma (metastatic).	Vemurafenib[5].	BRAF-inhibitors.
Melanoma (metastatic).	Dabrafenid[5].	BRAF-inhibitors.
Melanoma (metastatic).	Trametinib[5].	MEK inhibitors.

[1]Woodmansee C1, Pillow J, Skinner RB Jr.The role of topical immune response modifiers in skin cancer. *Drugs*. 2006;66:1657-64.

[2]Singh M, Khong H, Dai Z, Huang XF, Wargo JA, Cooper ZA et al. Effective innate and adaptive antimelanoma immunity through localized TLR7/8 activation. *J Immunol.* 2014;193:4722-1.

[3]Mashima E, Inoue A, Sakuragi Y, Yamaguchi T, Sasaki N, Hara Y et al. Nivolumab in the treatment of malignant melanoma: review of the literature. *Onco Targets Ther.* 2015;8:2045-1.

[4]Mahoney KM, Freeman GJ, McDermott DF. The Next Immune-Checkpoint Inhibitors: PD-1/PD-L1 Blockade in Melanoma. *Clin. Ther.* 2015;37:764-82.

[5]Niezgoda A, Niezgoda P, Czajkowski R. Novel Approaches to Treatment of Advanced Melanoma: A Review on Targeted Therapy and Immunotherapy. *Biomed. Res. Int.* 2015;2015:851387.

Oral Medicine for Advanced Basal Cell Carcinoma

Erivedge™ (vismodegib) was approved by the FDA in 2012 for extraordinarily rare cases of metastatic BCC or locally advanced BCC that become dangerous and even life-threatening [39] (Table 2). The first medicine ever for advanced BCC, it works by blocking the "Hedgehog" signaling pathway, which is a key step in the development of BCC. It is approved only for very limited circumstances where the nature of the cancer precludes other treatment options (such as surgery or radiation).

Several other targeted Hedgehog inhibitors are also being investigated as potential treatments for locally advanced and metastatic BCC. Due to a risk of birth defects, vismodegib should not be used by women who are pregnant or may become pregnant. Birth control must be used by couples if the woman is capable of becoming pregnant.

Immune Response to BCC

In this book we are presenting different chapters with case reports showing several type of immune response against BCC which we invite the readers to review. This immune response was seen in several cases with the presence of antigen presenting cells CD68 positive around the tumor and several T lymphocytes.

Keratoacanthomas: Actinic Cheilitis and Leuklopakia are Considering also as Precancers

The most common type of oral cancer is SCC, which accounts for about 90% of all oral malignancies. Therefore, the oral cancer problem primarily concerns the diagnosis, biology and management of SCC. However, there are red and white lesions that are considered premalignant, since they may unpredictably transform into cancer.

According to the (World Health Organization) leukoplakia, eritroplakia and actinic cheilitis are considered precancerous lesions which pathologically may correspond to intraepithelial dysplasia, hyperkeratosis, carcinoma in situ or SCC [40-46]. Kerathoacanthomas are more commonly associates with xerodermapigmentosum.

It is believed that the rate of the malignant transformation of premalignant lesion is about 32.6% for keratoacanthoma, 16.9% for actinic cheilitis, 10% for actinic keratoses. Some of these are commonly present in the lower lip possibly due to the UV radiation. In general clinical resection is the treatment of option because topical fluoracile could cause an extreme burn in those areas [40-46].

The infundibular keratinizing acanthoma (kerathoanahoma) is a rare epithelial benign keratin-containing neoplasm of hair follicles. A typical IKA consisted of a keratin-filled crypt in the dermis and subcutis that opened to the skin surface. Most of this tumor occurred on the back, neck, head, and the shoulders. Microscopically, the dermal nodules were focally contiguous in both the dermis and subcutis [40-42].

Furthermore, most histological lesions are consistent with a simple or multi-loculated cyst filled with keratin and lined by a wall of stratified squamous epithelium; keratin appears as a concentric lamellar mass, with a keratotic pearly aspects. Keratoacanthomas frequently show chromosomal aberrations as assessed by comparative genomic hybridization [40-42].

Leukoplakia

Oral and genital cancers arelinked to well-known behavioral risk factors such as tobacco smoking and alcohol consumption [43-45]. Other risk factors include age over 40, male sex, several dietary factors, nutritional deficiencies, viruses, sexually transmitted infections, human papillomavirus, chronic irritation, and possibly genetic predisposition. Precancerous lesions in the oral cavity include leukoplakia, erythroplakia, and lichen planus.

Histology of oral cancer varies widely but the great majorities are squamous cell carcinomas [43-45]. Epidemiological studies and cancer registries have shown a consistently increased risk of oral malignancies in kidney, bone marrow, heart, or liver transplantation, in graft vs host disease, and in patients with HIV infection.

Because of the increasing use of immunosuppressive drugs in patients with inflammatory bowel disease, it is useful to more accurately delineate the consequences of chronic immunosuppression to the oral cavity. Education on modifiable risk behaviors in patients with oral cancer is the cornerstone of prevention.Oral screening should be performed for all IBD patients, especially those who are about to start an immunosuppressant or biological drug [43-45].

Actinic Cheilitis

Actinic keratosis is the same name as actinic keratoses mentioned above [46].

Bowen's Disease

This is now generally considered an early, noninvasive stage of SCC. It appears as a persistent red-brown, scaly patch that may resemble psoriasis or eczema [47]. If untreated, it may invade deeper structures. Bowen's disease is most often caused by exposure to the sun or to arsenic, but radiation and other chemical carcinogens, genetics and trauma also may play a role. The human Papillomavirus (HPV), highly transmissible through sexual contact, has been documented as a cause of one form of Bowen's disease affecting the genitals. HPV can also arise in the mucous membranes of the nose and mouth as well as on the skin. The FDA approved an HPV vaccine for use by females aged 9–26 in 2006 and one for 9-26 year-old males (as well as another vaccine for females) in 2009. The vaccines areconsidered highly effective in preventing HPV and thereby reducing the risk of genital warts and cervical cancer as well as Bowen's disease (Figure 1) [47].

Squamous Cell Carcinomas (SCC)

SCC is at least twice as frequent in men as in women, partly because of more time spent in the sun. Most SCCs appear in people over 50, but in recent years more and more young people in their 20s and 30'sare being diagnosed with the disease. The number of women under age 40 diagnosed with SCC has especially increased in the last 30 years, and many experts attribute this to their greater use of indoor tanning. More than 419,000 cases of skin cancer in the US each year are linked to indoor tanning, and over 70 percent of tanning salon patrons is female. The majority of skin cancers in African-Americans are squamous cell carcinomas, usually arising on the sites of preexisting inflammatory skin conditions or burn injuries. Though naturally dark-skinned people are less likely than fair-skinned people to get skin cancer, it is still essential for them to practice sun protection. All skin types are at risk of skin cancer [48]. Recently, there has been a large increase in new SCCs diagnosed in Latinos and other people of color.

Cumulative exposure to sunlight causes most cases of squamous cell carcinoma. Frequent use of tanning beds also multiplies the risk of squamous cell carcinoma; people who use tanning beds are 2.5 times more likely to develop squamous cell carcinoma than those who don't. But skin injuries are another important source. The cancer can arise in burns, scars, ulcers, long-standing sores, and sites previously exposed to X-rays or certain chemicals (such as arsenic and petroleum by-products). Chronic infections and skin inflammation can also give rise to SCC.

Furthermore, human immunodeficiency virus (HIV) and other immune deficiency diseases, chemotherapy, anti-rejection drugs used in organ transplantation [49], and even excessive sun exposure itself all weaken the immune system, making it harder to fight off disease and thus increasing the risk of developing squamous cell carcinoma and other skin cancers. Studies have shown that organ transplant recipients are up to 250 times more likely than the general population to develop SCC.

Occasionally, SCC arises spontaneously on what appears to be normal, healthy skin. Some researchers believe the tendency to develop these cancers can be inherited. SCCthat isdetected at an early stage can be removed promptly, and are almost always curable and cause minimal damage. However, left untreated, they eventually penetrate the underlying tissues and can become disfiguring [50]. A small percentage even metastasizes to local lymph nodes, distant tissues, and organs, this can become fatal. Therefore, any suspicious growth should be seen by a physician without delay. A biopsy will be examined under a microscope to arrive at a diagnosis. If tumor cells are present, treatment is required.

Fortunately, there are several effective ways to eradicate SCC. The choice of treatment is based on the tumor's type, size, location, and depth of penetration, as well as the patient's age and general health. Treatment can almost always be performed on an outpatient basis in a physician's office or at a clinic. A local anesthetic is used during most surgical procedures. Pain or discomfort is usually minimal, and there is rarely much pain afterwards [50].

Treatment of SCC

Is similar to BCC. Definitely is better a large surgical excision or resectionwith good and ample deep and lateral margins (above the other treatments). In some case it does require lymph node dissections and histological and IHC studies of the dissected tissue for the putative metastasis [50] (Table 3).

Table 3. Most common immunohistochemical stains in skin and pre-skin cancers

Lesions	IHC stain	Targets
BCC	Ber-Ep4	
SCC	Pan cytokeratin antibodies. AE1/AE31 or Lu-5 antibodies	Pan cytokeratin antibodies for both acidic (type 1) and basic type (basic type 2) keratins.
SCC	High Molecular Weight Cytokeratin (HMW CK)[34βE12]2	
Dermatofibrosarcoma protuberans	CD34	
Melanoma, schwnomas	S100A	Antibody S100 stains melanocytes, schwannomas, peripheral neural tissue astrocytes, and benign and malignant melanomas and their metastases. Also express in Langerhans cells in skin and interdigitating reticulum cells in the paracortex of lymph nodes
Melanoma	MITF	Master regulator of melanocyte development and melanoma oncogene
Melanoma	SOX-10	It is a nuclear transcription factor that plays an important role in melanocytic cell differentiation.
Melanoma	HMB45	It is a neuraminidase-sensitive oligosaccharide side chain of a glycoconjugate, is present in immature melanosomes
Melanoma	MART-1/Melan A	It recognizes a protein of 18 kDa, identified at MART-1 (Melanoma Antigen Recognized by Tcells 1) or Melan-A. The MART-1 recognizes a subcellular fraction found in melanosomes. The antibody labels melanomas and tumors showing melanocytic differentiation

Lesions	IHC stain	Targets
Melanoma, desmoplastic melanomas	Tyrosine	It is s a key enzyme involved in the initial stages of melanin biosynthesis.
Langerhans cell histiocytosis.	CD1a	
Differentiate between dermatofibroma and dermatofibrosarcoma protuberans.	Factor XIII, CD34	
Adenocarcinomas	Low Molecular Weight Cytokeratin (LMW CK) Clone 5D3	It recognizes CK 8/18 intermediate filament proteins
T-cell lymphomas, including mycosis fungoides.	CD4	It is expressed in a T-cell subset (helper/inducer) and is found in approximately 80% of thymocytes and 45% of peripheral blood lymphocytes
Mycosis fungoides	CD7	It is molecule is a membrane-bound glycoprotein of 40kD, and is the earliest T-cell specific antigen to be expressed in lymphocytes. It is expressed in the majority of thymocytes, peripheral blood T cells, and natural killer cells.
Peripheral nerve sheath tumors and pheochromocytomas, neurotropic melanomas.	Nerve Growth Factor (p75) Monoclonal antibody NGFR, p75	NGFR reacts with peripheral nerve sheath tumors and pheochromocytomas. S
Merkel Cell Carcinoma	Neuroendrocrine and LMW cytokeratin, Chromogranin A or B, CK20	

Lentigomaligna, Dysplastic Nevus

These are the more common premalignant lesions to the development of melanoma. Lentigo maligna (LM) can histologically simulate dysplastic nevus (DN). Partial biopsy of LM may lead to misdiagnosis that can lead to devastating results.

Large pigmented lesions on sun-damaged skin in elderly individuals should warrant consideration of LM/LMM diagnosis, even in the setting of DN-like features histologically. Excisional biopsy may help to avoid misdiagnosis [51, 52].

Melanoma

Is the most deadly skin cancer, however if melanoma is recognized and treated promptly, it is nearly always curable, but if it is not, the cancer can advance and spread to other parts of the body, where it becomes more difficult to treat and can be deadly [53-56]. While it is not the most common of the skin cancers, it causes the majority of the deaths. The American Cancer Society estimates that at the present, more than 120,000 new cases of melanoma in the US are diagnosed in a year. In 2014, around 70,100 cases were foundto be invasive melanomas, with around 43,890 in males and 32,210 in women [53-56].

Melanoma Warning Signs

The "ABCDEs" of Melanoma. Moles, brown spots and growths on the skin are generally harmless, but not all the time. Anybody who has more than about 100 moles is at larger risk for melanoma [53-56]. The initial signs can look like one or more atypical moles. That's why it's so imperative to teach the patients at risk of melanoma and other skin cancer to know their skin, to do an examination of their skin using two mirrors at least every two months and to visit the dermatologist or a physician every three months to evaluate putative any changes in the "moles" [53-56]. The patients should look for the "ABCDE" signs of possible melanoma, and if changes are seen, the patients need to be instructed to make an appointment with a physician immediately [53-56].

Risk Factors for Melanoma

Everyone is at some risk for melanoma, but increased risk depends on several factors: sun exposure, number of moles on the skin, skin type and family history (genetics) [53-56].

Family History for Melanoma

Heredity plays a major role in melanoma. About one in every 10 patients diagnosed with the disease has a family member with a history of melanoma [53-54]. If your mother, father, siblings or children have had a melanoma, you are in a melanoma-prone family. Each person with a first-degree relative diagnosed with melanoma has a 50 percent greater chance of developing the disease than people who do not have a family history of the disease [53-56].

The Stages of Melanoma

Once the type of melanoma has been established, the next step is to classify the disease as to its degree of severity. Classifications for melanomas are called stages. The stage refers to the thickness, depth of penetration, and the degree to which the melanoma has spread [53-56]. The staging is used to determine treatment. Early melanomas (Stages 0 and I) are localized; Stage 0 tumors are in situ, meaning that they are noninvasive and have not penetrated below the surface of the skin, while Stage I tumors have invaded the skin but are small, nonulcerated, and are growing at a slow mitotic rate. Stage II tumors, though localized, are larger (generally over 1 mm. thick) and/or may be ulcerated or have a mitotic rate of greater than 1/mm2; they are considered intermediate melanomas [53-56]. More advanced melanomas (Stages III and IV) have spread (metastasized) to other parts of the body. There are also subdivisions within stages.

The Four Types of Melanomas

Three of them begin in situmeaning (in the skin), and sometimes become invasive; the fourth is invasive from the start. Invasive melanomas are more serious, as they have penetrated deeper into the skin and may have spread to other areas of the body [53-56].

Superficial Spreading Melanoma

It is the most common type, accounting for about 70 percent of all cases. This is the one most often seen in young people [53-56]. As the name suggests, this melanoma grows along the top layer of the skin for a fairly long time before penetrating deeper. The first sign is the appearance of a flat or slightly raised discolored patch that has irregular borders and is somewhat asymmetrical in form. The color varies, and you may see areas of tan, brown, black, red, blue or white [53-56]. This type of melanoma can occur in a previously benign mole. The melanoma can be found almost anywhere on the body, but is most likely to occur on the trunk in men, the legs in women, and the upper back in both.

Lentigo Maligna Melanoma

It is similar to the superficial spreading type, as it also remains close to the skin surface for quite a while, and usually appears as a flat or mildly elevated mottled tan, brown or dark brown discoloration [53-56]. This type of in situ melanoma is found most often in the elderly, arising on chronically sun-exposed, damaged skin on the face, ears, arms and upper trunk. Lentigo maligna is the most common form of melanoma in Hawaii. When this cancer becomes invasive, it is referred to as lentigo maligna melanoma [53-56].

Acral Lentiginous Melanoma

This form of melanoma also spreads superficially before penetrating deeper. It is quite different from the others, though, as it usually appears as a black or brown discoloration under the nails or on the soles of the feet or palms of the hands [53-56]. This type of melanoma is sometimes found on dark-skinned people, and can often advance more quickly than superficial spreading melanoma and lentigomaligna. It is the most common melanoma in African-Americans and Asians, and the least common among Caucasians [53-56].

Nodular Melanoma

Nodular melanoma is usually invasive at the time it is first diagnosed. The malignancy is recognized when it becomes a bump. It is usually black, but occasionally is blue, gray, white, brown, tan, red or skin tone [53-56]. The most frequent locations are the trunk, legs, and arms, mainly of elderly people, as well as the scalp in men. This is the most aggressive of the melanomas, and is found in 10 to 15 percent of cases [53-56].

IHC Stains for Melanoma

Several stains have been used to identify melanocytes when evaluating melanoma including S-100, human melanoma black-45 (HMB-45), melanoma 5 (Mel-5), and MART-1 (melanoma antigen recognized by T-cells 1 staining) also known as Melan-A [57, 58]. The utilization of stains is guided by the type of melanoma and the stain's sensitivity and specificity for melanoma. For example, S-100 staining remains the best diagnostic marker in desmoplastic and spindle cell melanoma [57, 58]. Furthermore, some authors reported that Melan-A was the most reliable stain for melanoma while HMB-45 appeared to be the least consistent stain. Histological evaluation of epidermal melanocytes on routine staining is difficult and cannot be made with accuracy [57, 58]. Widely known antibodies such as S-100 and HMB-45 are unreliable for normal epidermal melanocytes. Furthermore, S-100 stains other cells including Langerhans' cells [57, 58]. Results of incubation with DOPA are inconsistent and the procedure is time-consuming (Table 3).

HMB-45

HMB-45 is a proliferative marker that recognizes glycoprotein 100 in immature melanosomes. Immature melanosomes are found in growing, undeveloped melanocytes, and are characteristic of melanoma [57, 58] (Table 3). However, immature melanosomes are also found in benign melanocytic lesions, inflammatory skin conditions, skin over vascular structures and near scar tissue, and neonatal skin. While HMB-45 may be specific for melanocytic tumors, it has lacked consistent sensitivity in the detection of melanomas. It has been reported that HMB-45 stained positively in only 85 percent of all melanoma cases and offered a slight advantage of decreased background staining due to HMB-45's lack of keratinocyte affinity.35 HMB-45 has been found to be more specific than S-100 for melanocytic lesions but inconsistent with identifying desmoplastic melanomas [57, 58]. In addition, while HMB-45 correctly identifies most melanomas, it has failed to stain isolated areas of in situ and invasive melanocytic proliferations that were recognized by other immunestains.

S-100

S-100 is the most important historical stain for melanoma. It is a polyclonal antibody to a protein derived from cow brain [57, 58]. The S-100 molecule consists of two subunits—an alpha unit that reacts with axons and melanocytes and a beta unit that reacts with Schwann cells [57].

S100 stains almost all benign melanocytic lesions as well as a variety of other tissues including salivary and sweat glands, dendritic cells, skeletal and cardiac muscle, histiocytes, chondrocytes and lipocytes. S-100 remains the stain of choice for evaluating desmoplastic and spindle cell melanoma, but is less reliable than (HMB-45, Mel-5, and Melan A) in recognizing epidermal melanocytic proliferation. However, S-100 has maintained its superiority in identifying the dermal component of melanomas [57, 58].

Mel-5

Histological differentiation between pigmented actinic keratosis in photodamaged skin and lentigo maligna can be problematic. The atypical keratinocytes, particularly in the basal layer, can be confused with atypical melanocytes, particularly if they are pigmented [59].

Likewise, differences between lichen planus-like keratosis and lichenoid melanoma in situ and lentigo maligna and lentigo may be problematic. Use of Mel-5 in such cases has shown reliable results in separating melanocytic from non-melanocytic lesions. This antibody is also helpful in evaluating biopsies of patients with vitiligo, post-inflammatory pigmentary alteration and regressed or regressing melanocytic lesions. Furthermore, Mel-5 is a priceless tool in quantification of epidermal melanocytes [59, 60].

PNL2 in Melanoma

PNL2 is a monoclonal antibody used to stain melanocyte and tumors derived [59, 60]. Some authors analyzed the immunoreactivity of this antibody in various normal tissues, melanocytic nevi, primary and metastatic melanoma, nonmelanocytic tumors, including histologic mimickers of melanoma as well as angiomyolipoma, and multiple cell lines derived from different tumors types. For metastatic melanoma, immunoreactivity for PNL2 was compared with A103 (Melan-A/MART-1), T311 (tyrosinase), HMB45 (gp100), and D5 (MITF) [59, 60].

Positive staining with PNL2 was found in normal melanocytes and neutrophils, but no other normal cell type. Among melanocytic lesions, both benign nevi as well as primary malignant melanomas, especially epithelioid variants thereof, were commonly immunopositive. Only 1 in 13 desmoplastic melanomas reacted with PNL2 [ ].

The authors reported that PNL2 showed high sensitivity for metastatic melanoma (87%) in contrast, 82% of metastatic melanomas were positive for A103, 76% for HMB45, 92% for T311, and 84% for D5 [59, 60].

Nonmelanocytic tumors (carcinomas or soft tissue neoplasms) was positive for PNL2 in this series except for angiomyolipomas and chronic myeloid leukemias and 1 single case of a malignant peripheral nerve sheath tumor with heterologous differentiation (malignant Triton tumor) [59, 60].

Despite its reactivity with neutrophils, PNL2 appears to be a valuable supplementary reagent for the diagnosis of melanocytic tumors. The authors didn't study any amelanotyc melanoma.

Treatment for Melanoma

The first step in treatment is the removal of the melanoma, and the standard method of doing this is by surgical excision (cutting it out). Surgery has made great advances in the past decade, and much less tissue is removed than was customary in the past [61-63]. Patients do just as well after the laser surgery, which is easier to tolerate and produces a smaller scar.Surgical excision is also called resection, and the borders of the entire area excised are known as the margins [61-63].

Outpatient/Office Surgery

In most cases, the surgery for thin melanomas can be done in the doctor's office or as an outpatient procedure under local anesthesia. Stitches (sutures) remain in place for one to two weeks, and most patients are advised to avoid heavy exercise during this time [61-63]. Scars are usually small and improve over time.Discolorations and areas that are depressed or raised following the surgery can be concealed with cosmetics specially formulated to provide camouflage [61-63]. If the melanoma is larger and requires more extensive surgery, a better cosmetic appearance can be obtained with flaps made from skin near the tumor, or with grafts of skin taken from another part of the body. For grafting, the skin is removed from areas that are normally or easily covered with clothing.There is now a trend towards performing sentinel node biopsy and tumor removal surgery at the same time provided the tumor is 1 mm or thicker [61-63]. When the procedures are combined in this way, the patient is spared an extra visit.Surgical excision or resection: o called resection, and the borders of the entire area excised are known as the margins. Surgical excision is used to treat all types of skin cancer. At its best - given an experienced surgeon and a small, well-placed tumor - it offers results that are both medically and cosmetically excellent [61-63]. The physician begins by outlining the tumor with a marking pen [61-63]. A "safety margin" of healthy-looking tissue will be included, because it is not possible to determine with the naked eye how far microscopic strands of tumor may have extended.

The extended line of excision is drawn, so the skin may be sewn back together. The physician will administer a local anesthetic, and then cut along the lines that were drawn. The entire procedure may take about thirty minutes for smaller lesions [61-63].

The skin wounds usually heal rapidly, (between one to three weeks). The presence of scarring depends on many factors, includingthe placement of the tumor, the patient's care of the wound after the procedure and genetic factors intrinsic to each person [61-63].

The sample that was taken is examined in a frozen cut at minus 20 centigrade in a cryostat to see if the sample has margins that are free of tumor. If the margins are not free, and additional surgery is required.

Setting the Margins

In the new approach to surgery, much less of the normal skin around the tumor is removed and the margins, therefore, are much narrower than they ever were before. This spares significant amounts of tissue and reduces the need for postoperative cosmetic reconstructive surgery [61-63].

Most US surgeons today follow the guidelines recommended by the National Institutes of Health and the American Academy of Dermatology Task Force on Cutaneous Melanoma. When there is an in situ melanoma, the surgeon excises 0.5-1 centimeter of the normal skin surrounding the tumor and takes off the skin layers down to the fat. In removing an invasive melanoma that is 1 mm or less in Breslow's thickness, the margins of surrounding skin are extended to 1 cm and the excision goes through all skin layers and down to the fascia (the layer of tissue covering the muscles). If the melanoma is 1.01 to 2 mm thick, a margin of 1-2 cm is taken. If the melanoma is 2.01 mm thick or greater, a margin of 2 cm is taken [61-63].

These margins all fall within the range of what is called "narrow" excision. When you consider that until recently, margins of 3 to 5 cm (wide excision) were standard, even for comparatively thin tumors, you can see how dramatically surgery has changed for the better.

Physicians now know that even when melanomas have reached a thickness of 4 mm or more, increasing the margin beyond 2 cm does not increase survival [61-63].

Familial Melanoma Syndrome (FM)

Initially titled familial atypical multiple mole melanoma (FAMMM) syndrome, with early descriptions of augmented hyperdiploidy observed as an in vitro phenomenon in cultured skin fibroblasts from high-risk and affected subjects [64, 65]. The FAMMM genotype was defined as complex in that it predisposed a patient not only to melanoma (cutaneous and intraocular malignant melanoma) but also to other kinds of cancer including lung, pancreas, and breast [24, 64, 65]. After recognizing this entity, care was initially focused on cancer surveillance and management programs for patients at increased risk for the several forms of hereditary FM [24, 64, 65]. Genetic analysis done long ago in some families with clinical and pathologic verification of the FAM syndrome had shown some at peril members in these families, with a segregation ratio of about 0.47 (dependable with an autosomal dominant mode of inheritance) [24, 64, 65]. Some obligate gene carriers who lacked any FM phenotypic manifestations were observed, and the rate of penetrance for the FM gene was calculated to be 0.93.

Microphthalmia-Associated Transcription Factor (MITF)

MITF in melanoma acts as a master regulator of melanocyte development, function and survival by modulating various differentiation and cell-cycle progression genes. It is a great IHC stain for melanoma (Table 3). It has been demonstrated that MITF is an amplified oncogene in a fraction of human melanomas and that it also has an oncogenic role in human clear cell sarcoma. However, MITF also modulates the state of melanocyte differentiation. A malignant neoplasm of melanocytes, arising either from pre-existing benign nevi or de novo and occurring most commonly on the skin, but may occur in other locations. There have been linkage and genome wide association studies (GWAS) studies that have shown no indication to implicate MITF in melanoma [24, 66]. However, MITF has been shown to be mutated in a subset of melanomas and overexpressed in others. This raises the possibility of MITF's involved despite the lack of prior indication for germline risk. Indeed, individuals with a specific MITF mutation (E318K) have a 5-fold increase risk of developing melanoma [24, 66]. MITF amplification has also been associated with decreased survival and chemoresistance. It is hypothesized the MITF may be a lineage specific oncogene in melanoma, particularly in the subset with CDKN2A mutations [24, 66].

This hypothesis is supported by research that has shown that all melanoma cell lines that had MITF gene amplifications also had CDKN2A pathway inactivation. MITFs role as a lineage specific oncogene is also maintained by its important part in cell growth, survival, growth, and proliferation through BCL2, CDK2, TBX2, ML-IAP [24, 66, 67].

In addition, BRAF mutations is found in ~60% of melanomas and have a two-fold regulation of MITF transcription and is supposed to keep MITF at suitable levels promoting melanoma cell proliferation and survival.

Backing up this theory is the fact that pure up-regulation of MITF inhibits melanoma cell proliferation and re-expression reduces tumorigenecity *in vivo*. Other altered genes in melanoma that has been show to play a genetic role seem to be metalloproteinase enzymes 8 [24].

Sry-Related HMg-Box Gene 10 (SOX10)

Itis a nuclear transcription factor that plays an important role in melanocytic cell differentiation. SOX10 in melanoma (Table 3). SOX10 is a transcription factor located at 22q13.1, locusID (NCBI) 6663, starts at 38368319 and ends at 38380539 bp from pter. SOX10Location_base_pair is flanked by POLR2F (DNA-directed RNA polymerase II polypeptide F) and PICK1 (protein interacting with PRKCA.

This genes mutation has been often described in melanoma. This gene was first identified as a gene mutated in patients suffering from Waardenburg syndrome type 4C (WS4C) [68, 69]. SOX10 mutations also cause Waardenburg syndrome type 2E (WS2E) with or without neurologic involvement, Yemenite deaf-blind hypopigmentation syndrome and PCWH syndrome. They usually occur in the heterozygous state and can be either sporadic or familial [68, 69].

All 20 human members of this protein family possess a high-mobility-group (HMG) domain with three alpha-helical regions and close similarity to the one found in the male sex determining factor Khong HT, Rosenberg SA. The Waardenburg syndrome type 4 gene, SOX10, is a novel tumor-associated antigen identified in a patient with a dramatic response to immunotherapy. The A newly developed mouse monoclonal SOX10 antibody.

V-Raf Murine Sarcoma Viral Oncogene Homolog B1 (BRAF) in Melanoma

BRAF locusID (NCBI) is 673, its location is 7q34, and its location_base _pair starts at 140433813 and ends at 140624564 bp from pter and it local order is between the NDUFB2 and MRPS33 genes [24, 70]. BRAF is a serine/threonine kinase that belongs to the RAS/RAF/MEK/ERK/MAPK pathway, which is involved in the transduction of mitogenic signals from the cell membrane to the nucleus. RAS is inactive when binded to GDP, but when it binds to GTP becomes active and promotes phosphorylation and activation of BRAF and the activation of the pathway signal [24, 70]. Several genes have been found to be activated by this pathway, among them, cyclin D1, cyclin D2 and cyclin D3 (self-sufficiency in growth), VEGF (angiogenesis), c-myc (insensitivity to anti-growth signals), b3-integrin (tissue invasion and metastasis) and mdm2 (apoptosis evasion, limitless replicative potential and angiogenesis). BRAF is mutated in 70% of malignant melanomas [24, 70].

Immune Therapy for Melanoma

Topical Imiquimod (IQ)

It is an effective treatment for genital warts and various malignant tumors of the skin. IQ acts through the Toll-like receptor 7 leading to the production of cytokines and chemokines such as interferons, interleukins, and growth factors. Immunophenotyping revealed in all cases during treatment and increased population of T-lymphocytes positive for CD3, CD4 and CD8, as well as a considerable number of cytotoxic cells (TIA-1+, granzyme B+) and plasmacytoid dendritic cells (CD 123+). These findings further support previous investigations that the antitumor effects of IQ result from an enhanced cytotoxic T-cell mediated immune response and from the recruitment of plasmacytoid dendritic cells to the skin. The population of infiltrative inflammatory cells was similar in all patients irrespective of the type of tumor [71]. T cell-mediated immunity to microbes and to cancer can be enhanced by the activation of dendritic cells (DCs) via TLRs. In this study, we evaluated the safety and feasibility of topical imiquimod, a TLR7 agonist, in a series of vaccinations against the cancer/testis Ag NY-ESO-1 in patients with malignant melanoma.

Recombinant, full-length NY-ESO-1 protein was administered intradermally into imiquimod preconditioned sites followed by additional topical applications of imiquimod.

Mohs Surgery

It is not recommended for melanoma for fear that some microscopic melanoma cells might be missed and end up metastasizing.

Some Important Concepts to Know in Skin and Pre-Skin Cancers

In Situ Immunization

It is based on the concept that it is possible to break immune tolerance by inducing tumor cell death in situ in a manner that provides antigen-presenting cells such as dendritic cells with a wide selection of tumor antigens that can then be presented to the immune system and result in a therapeutic anticancer immune response.

Oncogenes and Tumor Suppressor Genes

Two of the main types of genes that play a role in cancer are oncogenes and tumor suppressor genes (TSG). Oncogenes Proto-oncogenes are genes that normally help cells grow. When a proto-oncogene mutates (changes) or there are too many copies of it, it becomes a corrupt gene that can become permanently turned on or activated when it should not be. When this happens, the cell grows out of control, which can lead to cancer [24].

This bad gene is called an oncogene. A few cancer syndromes are caused by inherited mutations of proto-oncogenes that cause the oncogene to be activated. But most cancer-causing mutations involving oncogenes are acquired (somatic mutations), not inherited. They generally activate oncogenes by several mechanism such chromosome rearrangements that changes in chromosomes that put one gene next to another, which allows one gene to activate the other and also by gene duplication in TSG [24].

TSG are normal genes that slow down cell division, repair DNA mistakes, or tell cells when to die (apoptosis). When TSG doesn't work properly, cells can grow out of control, which can lead to cancer. When something goes wrong with the gene, such as a mutation, cell division can get out of control. An important difference between oncogenes and TSG, is that oncogenes result from the activation (turning on) of proto-oncogenes, but TSG cause cancer when they are inactivated (turned off). Inherited abnormalities of TSG have been found in some family cancer syndromes [24]. Finding certain genes or gene mutations can be helpful in diagnosing skin cancer, monitoring the effects of treatment, learning about prognosis, and in treating of skin cancer [24].

Genes and Skin Cancer Prognosis

In some cancers, specific gene changes can be used to predict which patients are likely to have a better or worse outcome. This can help guide the intensity of treatment. For some cancers, tests that look at the activity (expression) of many genes at once can be useful in predicting prognosis [72]. These tests, called gene expression panels, are performed on samples of the cancer. Drugs have been developed that target some of the gene changes in certain cancers. Actually, these drugs often target the protein made by the abnormal gene (and not the gene itself) [73]. Drugs targeting certain mutations are useful in a number of other cancers and melanoma. Drugs that activate genes DNA methylation is one way to turn-off genes. Drugs called hypomethylating agents can reverse methylation. This can be helpful in treating some cancers in which some genes are abnormally methylated. Some hypomethylatingagent'sdecitabine (Dacogen®) and azacytidine (Vidaza®) can decrease this abnormal methylation, which can be useful in treating this disease. Other drugs that help fight cancer by activating genes are the histone deacetylase inhibitors [72]. Other treatments include *in situ* immunization, based on the concept that it is possible to break immune tolerance by inducing tumor cell death in situ in a manner that provides antigen-presenting cells such as dendritic cells (DCs). This is theorically possible by using a wide selection of tumor antigens that can then be presented to the immune system and result in a therapeutic anticancer immune response [73]. Some authors had described in situ immunization using poly(lactic-co-glycolic acid) (PLGA)-biodegradable microparticles (MPs) loaded with doxorubicin (Dox) and CpGoligodeoxynucleotides (CpG) that deliver Dox (chemotherapy) and CpG (immunotherapy) in a sustained-release fashion when injected intratumorally. The authors claim that the combination regimen is effective at reducing T cell lymphoma and melanoma tumor burdens and conclude that Dox/CpG MPs represent an efficient and safe tool for in situ immunization that could provide a promising component of immunotherapy for patients with a variety of types of cancer [73].

Carney Complex (CC)

It is a familial multiple neoplasia and lentiginosis syndrome, transmitted in an autosomal dominant (AD) manner. It is the single familial form of cardiac and skin myxomas known and includes endocrine neoplasms causing Cushing's syndrome and acromegaly. The molecular defect leading to CC remains unknown, but was recently mapped to chromosome 2p16 by linkage analysis [24, 74, 75]. Some authors studied tumors and tumor cell lines from patients with CC demonstrating significant genomic, but not microsatellite length, instability [24, 74, 75].

Skin Schwannoma

Schwannomatosis is a rare form of neurofibromatosis (NF) that has only recently been documented and appears to affect around 1:40,000 individuals. As with NF1 and NF2, schwannomatosis may vary greatly between patients. Because of this, and because the population of individuals is so small and the disorder so recently characterized, these patients have, until recently, been hard to conclusively identify [76]. Some schuanomas are amelanotic and can be part of the Carney Syndrome [77]. People with schwannomatosis develop multiple schwannomas on cranial, spinal and peripheral nerves--but they do not develop vestibular tumors and do not go deaf. They also do not develop any other kinds of tumors (for example, meningiomas, ependymomas or astrocytomas) and do not have learning disabilities. People with schwannomatosis have problems with chronic pain that often exceeds their neurological problems. The first symptom of schwannomatosis is almost always pain, which can occur in any part of the body. Both schwannomas and neurofibromas originate in the insulating covering of peripheral nerves called the nerve sheath. Schwannomas are very homogenous tumors consisting exclusively of nerve sheath cells or Schwann cells [76].

They stay on the outside of the nerve, but may push it aside or against a bony structure causing damage. Diagnostic criteria for schwannomatosis: 1) Individual is age over 30 years, and has two or more non-intradermal schwannomas, at least one with histological confirmation, and has no evidence of vestibular tumor on high-quality MRI scan, and has no known constitutional NF2 mutation. or: Has one pathologically confirmed non-vestibular schwannoma plus a first-degree relative who meets the above criteria. Other possible additional diagnostic criteria for Schwannomatosis is to see an individual less than 30 years, and has two or more non-intradermal schwannomas, at least one with histological confirmation, and no evidence of vestibular tumor on high quality MRI scan, and no known constitutional NF2 mutation, or: Individual is age over 45 years, and has two or more non-intradermal schwannomas, at least one with histological confirmation, and has no symptoms of 8th cranial nerve dysfunction, and has no known constitutional NF2 mutation, or has radiographic evidence of a non-vestibular schwannoma and first degree relative meeting criteria for definite schwannomatosis [76].

Diagnostic Criteria for Segmental Schwannomatosis

Individuals who meet the above diagnostic criteria (or proposed diagnostic criteria) for schwannomatosis but this is limited to one limb, or to five or fewer contiguous segments of the spine [76].

Neurofibromas

Neurofibromas are very heterogeneous tumors, which incorporate all sorts of cells and structural elements in addition to the Schwann cells. They infiltrate the nerve and splay apart the individual nerve fibers. Neurofibromas, the most common tumors in NF, are benign growths which typically develop on or just underneath the surface of the skin but may also occur in deeper areas of the body [78-81]. Neurofibromas, which are composed of tissue from the nervous system (neuro) and fibrous tissue (fibroma), usually develop around puberty although they may appear at any age [78-81]. The tumors are not contagious. Nodule-like surface tumors are known as dermal neurofibromas. Plexiform neurofibromas grow diffusely under the skin surface or in deeper areas of the body [78-81]. The presence of multiple neurofibromas is an important diagnostic sign of NF. A single neurofibroma may occasionally occur in people who do not have NF. The number of neurofibromas varies widely among affected individuals from only a few to thousands. Dermal neurofibromas rarely, if ever, become cancerous. Such a change, called a malignant transformation, may occur, although very rarely, in plexiform tumors [78-81]. Some neurofibromas, depending on their location and size, can be removed surgically if they become painful or infected, or cosmetically troublesome. There is no evidence that removal of growths will increase the rate of appearance of new growths, or can cause incompletely removed tumors to change from benign to cancerous. Café-au-lait spots, the most common sign of NF, are the flat, pigmented spots on the skin, which are called by the French term for coffee (café) with milk (lait) because of their light tan color. In darker-skinned people, café-au-lait spots appear darker in color than surrounding skin [78-81]. People with NF almost always have six or more café-au-lait spots. (Fewer café-au-lait spots may occur in people who do not have NF; in fact, about 10% of the general population has one or two café-au-lait spots). The size of the spots that identify NF varies from 1/4 inch (5 mm) in children and 3/4 inch (15 mm) in adults to several inches in diameter or larger. In general, with few exceptions, tumors are not more likely to appear where there are spots [78-81]. Café-au-lait spots are usually present at birth in children who have NF or, generally, appear by two years of age. Iris nevi (also called Lisch nodules) are clumps of pigment in the colored part of the eye (iris). Iris nevi, which usually appear around puberty, can be distinguished from iris freckles (commonly seen in people without NF) by a simple and painless procedure called a slit-lamp examination, which is typically performed by an ophthalmologist. Iris nevi do not cause medical problems and do not affect vision. The presence of iris nevi can occasionally be helpful in confirming the diagnosis of NF [78-81].

Neurofibromatoses Diagnosis

The patient should have two or more of the following criteria, provided that no other disease accounts for the finding: family history of NF1, 6 or more light brown ("cafe-au-lait") spots on the skin, presence of two or more pea-sized bumps (neurofibromas) on the skin or one or more plexiform neurofibroma (larger areas on the skin that look swollen), freckling under the arms or in the groin area, pigmented bumps on the eye's iris (Lisch nodules), skeletal abnormalities such as tibial dysplasia (bowing of the legs), or thinning of the shin bone, tumor on the optic nerve that may interfere with vision, epilepsy. According to the most widely quoted NF studies, epilepsy in NF1 occurs with a frequency of 3.5-7.3%. The seizures associated with NF1 do not differ from seizures seen in the general population and, when not associated with a brain lesion, are generally well controlled with routine antiepileptic medications. The "phakomatosis" concept was formulated early in the twentieth century by the ophthalmologist van der Hoeve. He included 3 disorders in the group-neurofibromatosis, tuberous sclerosis complex, and von Hippel-Lindau syndrome--on the basis of the occurrence of patchy ophthalmologic manifestations in each disorder. Since the name was coined, much has been learned about the pathogenesis of these 3 disorders. It is clear that 2 of them--neurofibromatosis and tuberous sclerosis--are collective terms for multiple disorders. Each of the conditions are caused by distinct genetic defects, with little commonality in terms of protein function. Yet, in some respects, the disorders share a pathogenetic mechanism, that of the tumor suppressor gene. This review will briefly describe these disorders in light of what has been learned about underlying molecular pathogenesis. In each case, genetic testing is beginning to be available; principles of the use of genetic tests will be described. Laboratory tests are now available in most cases to determine whether a person has NF 1 or 2. Gene linkage testing is available for families with NF1 and NF2. Direct gene testing is currently available for NF1 and may be available for NF2 in the near future. These tests may be used for presymptomatic diagnosis. To find out whether you qualify for such tests, consult your nearest NF clinic or center. Occasionally, the signs of NF are not easy to identify. For example, café-au-lait spots may be so pale that they are not noticeable in ordinary light. For this reason, members of families in which NF has occurred are often concerned about whether they may have the NF gene, even if they have no obvious signs of the disorder. An examination by a physician familiar with the signs of NF is the best way currently available to determine whether NF is present. Examination of the skin may be helped by use of an ultraviolet light (Wood's lamp) which can occasionally identify very light café-au-lait spot pigmentation and can also help to differentiate this from pigmentation due to fungal infections of the skin. An examination that reveals no signs of NF can be considered reassuring, since it is extremely rare for an individual to inherit the gene and to show no detectable sign of the disorder. Some complications of NF1 are disfigurement, scoliosis, learning disabilities, large heads, optic gliomas, congenital defects of bone, hypertension, early or late onset of puberty, problems with growth (too short or too tall), mental retardation, higher risk for certain rare malignant tumors that occur in the brain, nerves or spinal cord, but probably have the same risk for "common" cancers (such as lung, breast, stomach, etc.) as the general population. Other possible complications are stroke, and itching of the skin Genetics Testing for NF1 Medical Genomics Laboratory at University of Alabama, Birmingham: Patients and families interested in direct gene testing for NF1 can contact the Medical Genomics Laboratory at UAB, phone (205) 934-5562. More information on testing is available at the MGL website.

Skin Neuromas, Perineuromas Andcutaneous Hyperneury

Skin neuromas usually are solitary, circumscribed neuroma and are in general distinctive benign cutaneous tumors that were first described under the name "palisaded, encapsulated neuroma" over 15 years ago [82]. These lesions practically always present on the face or close to a mucocutaneous junction in middle-aged adults. Most examples measure less than or equal to 0.5 cm and are composed of a partially encapsulated mass of bland Schwann cells and multiple tiny axons arranged in interlacing fascicles [82]. The capsule is composed of perineural cells that show epithelial membrane antigen positivity. Solitary, circumscribed neuroma is not associated with von Recklinghausen's neurofibromatosis, nor is there evidence to support its possible relationship to the type IIb multiple endocrine neoplasia syndromes [82]. Because the multiples components of the nerves, many types of mixed neoplasias have been described with skin manifestation, some being very rare, some just being recognized as new entities [83-86]. Some of these entities are very rare skin neoplasias; some are completely asymptomatic some can cause hyperneury. Some are skincolored, some can be yellowish, with a linear or other shape patterns such a "bump" and or plaques/papules, most commonly described on the trunk and forearms and in general are of slow growing. Histological findings depends of the type of cells that originate the tumor and some may or not be associated with endocrine neoplasia type 2b [82-86].

Dermatofibrosarcoma Protuberans

Pigmented dermatofibrosarcomaprotuberance (DSFP) is a rare variant of DSFP. It isalso known as Bednar tumor or formerly known as Bednar first described it in 1957. The histology is striking because of the presence of multipolar pigment laden dendritic cells scattered among spindle shaped cells with a storiform pattern, the latter being characteristic of DSFP [87].

The spindle cells are positive for CD34 and vimentin and negative for S100. The similarity between the ultrastructure of the tumor cells and normal fibroblasts suggests the fibroblastic origin of the tumor. The pigment represents melanin. In patients with this tumor it is recommend doing a CT scan of chest, abdomen and pelvis.

Surgical excision with large margins and often reconstruction and/or full thickness skin transplantation is need [87-89]. Some authors have described non pigmented dermatofibrosarcoma protuberance.

Pleomorphic Dermal Sarcoma (PDS)

It is a rare neoplasm sharing pathological features with atypical fibroxanthoma, but adding tumor necrosis, invasion beyond superficial subcutis or vascular or perineural infiltration [90]. Metastatic risk is possible a lymph nodes and lungs and the lesions are in general tumors or plaques on the head of seniors, without gender predominance [90]. Histopathologically, they have spindle cells arranged in a fascicular pattern, containing pleomorphic epithelioid and giant multinucleated cells in varying proportions, and usually exhibiting numerous mitotic figures and infiltrative tumor margins. Cytokeratins, S100 protein, desmin or CD34 are usually positive, and necrosis and venous invasion can occur [90].

Other skin tumors like lymphomas are beyond the scope of this chapter.

Conflicts of interest

None.

Funding

Georgia Dermatopathology Associates, Atlanta, Georgia, US.

REFERENCES

[1] Criscione, V. D., Weinstock, M. A., Naylor, M. F., Luque, C., Eide, M. J., Bingham, S. F. Actinic keratoses: Natural history and risk of

malignant transformation in the Veterans Affairs Topical Tretinoin Chemoprevention Trial. *Cancer* 2009; 115:2523.

[2] Quaedvlieg, P. J., Tirsi, E., Thissen, M. R., Krekels, G. A. Actinic keratosis: how to differentiate the good from the bad ones? *Eur. J. Dermatol.* 2006; 16:335.

[3] Fuchs, A., Marmur, E. The kinetics of skin cancer: progression of actinic keratosis to squamous cell carcinoma. *Dermatol. Surg.* 2007; 33:1099.

[4] Jadotte, Y. T., Schwartz, R. A. Solar cheilosis: an ominous precursor: part I. Diagnostic insights. *J. Am. Acad. Dermatol.* 2012; 66:173.

[5] Thompson, S. C., Jolley, D., Marks, R. Reduction of solar keratoses by regular sunscreen use. *N. Engl. J. Med.* 1993; 329:1147.

[6] Marks, R., Rennie, G., Selwood, T. S. Malignant transformation of solar keratoses to squamous cell carcinoma. *Lancet* 1988; 1:795.

[7] Flohil, S. C., van der Leest, R. J., Dowlatshahi, E. A. et al. Prevalence of actinic keratosis and its risk factors in the general population: the Rotterdam Study. *J. Invest. Dermatol.* 2013; 133:1971.

[8] Salasche, S. J. Epidemiology of actinic keratoses and squamous cell carcinoma. *J. Am. Acad. Dermatol.* 2000; 42:4.

[9] Memon, A. A., Tomenson, J. A., Bothwell, J., Friedmann, P. S. Prevalence of solar damage and actinic keratosis in a Merseyside population. *Br. J. Dermatol.* 2000; 142:1154.

[10] Padilla, R. S., Sebastian, S., Jiang, Z., Nindl, I., Larson, R. Gene expression patterns of normal human skin, actinic keratosis, and squamous cell carcinoma: a spectrum of disease progression. *Arch. Dermatol.* 2010; 146:288.

[11] Ulrich, M., Drecoll, U., Stockfleth, E. Emerging drugs for actinic keratosis. *Expert Opin. Emerg. Drugs*. 2010;15:545-55.

[12] Stockfleth, E. Topical management of actinic keratosis and field cancerisation. *G. Ital. Dermatol. Venereol.* 2009;144:459-62.

[13] Isoherranen, K., Koskenmies, S., Overmark, M., Ylitalo, L., Saksela, O., Pitkänen, S. [Diagnosis and treatment of actinic keratosis]. *Duodecim.* 2015;131:863-70.

[14] Costa, C., Scalvenzi, M., Ayala, F., Fabbrocini, G., Monfrecola, G. How to treat actinic keratosis? An update. *J. Dermatol Case Rep.* 2015; 30;9: 29-35.

[15] Robinson, J. K. Current histologic preparation methods for Mohs Micrographic Surgery. *Dermatol. Surg.* 2001;27:555-60.

[16] Jimenez, F. J., Grichnik, J. M., Buchanan, M. D., Clark, R. E. Immunohistochemical techniques in Mohs micrographic surgery: their

potential use in the detection of neoplastic cells masked by inflammation. *J. Am. Acad. Dermatol.* 1995;32: 89-94.
[17] Zachary, C. B., Rest, E. B., Furlong, S. M., Arcedo, P. N., McGeorge, B. C., Kist, D. A. Rapid cytokeratin stains enhance the sensitivity of Mohs micrographic surgery for squamous cell carcinoma. *J. Dermatol. Surg. Oncol.* 1994;20:530-35.
[18] Mondragon, R. M., Barrett, T. L. Current concepts: the use of immunoperoxidase techniques in Mohs micrographic surgery. *J. Am. Acad. Dermatol.* 2000;43:66-71.
[19] Krunic, A. L., Garrod, D. R., Viehman, G. E., Madani, S., Buchanan, M. D., Clark, R. E. The use of antidesmoglein stains in Mohs micrographic surgery. A potential aid for the differentiation of basal cell carcinoma from horizontal sections of the hair follicle and folliculocentric basaloid proliferation. *Dermatol. Surg.* 1997;23:463-68.
[20] Smeets, N. W., Stavast-Kooy, A. J., Krekels, G. A., Daemen, M. J., Neumann, H. A. Adjuvant cytokeratin staining in Mohs micrographic surgery for basal cell carcinoma. *Dermatol. Surg.* 2003;29:375-77.
[21] Wells, J. W. Do actinic keratoses and superficial squamous cell carcinomas have a specific immunoprofile? *Curr. Probl. Dermatol.* 2015;46:36-41.
[22] Ulrich, C., Jürgensen, J. S., Degen, A. et al. Prevention of non-melanoma skin cancer in organ transplant patients by regular use of a sunscreen: a 24 months, prospective, case-control study. *Br. J. Dermatol.* 2009; 161 Suppl. 3:78.
[23] Marzuka, A. G., Book, S. E. Basal cell carcinoma: pathogenesis, epidemiology, clinical features, diagnosis, histopathology, and management. *Yale J. Biol. Med.* 2015;88:167-79.
[24] Abreu Velez, A. M., Howard, M. S. Tumor-suppressor Genes, Cell Cycle Regulatory Checkpoints, and the Skin. *N. Am. J. Med. Sci.* 2015;7: 176-88.
[25] Farndon, P. A., Del Mastro, R. G., Evans, D. G., Kilpatrick, M. W. Location of gene for Gorlinsyndrome. *Lancet.* 1992;339:581-82.
[26] Reis, A., Kuster, W., Linss, G., Gebel, E., Hamm, H., Fuhrmann, W. et al. Localisation of gene for the naevoid basal-cell carcinoma syndrome. *Lancet.* 1992;339:617.
[27] Gailani, M. R., Leffell, D. J., Ziegler, A., Gross, E. G., Brash, D. E., Bale, A. E. Relationship between sunlight exposure and a key genetic alteration in basal cell carcinoma. *J. Natl. Cancer Inst.* 1996;88:349-54.

[28] Hahn, H., Wicking, C., Zaphiropoulous, P. G., Gailani, M. R., Shanley, S., Chidambaram, A. et al. Mutations of the human homolog of Drosophila patched in the nevoid basal cell carcinoma syndrome. *Cell.* 1996;85:841-51.

[29] Altamura, D., Menzies, S. W., Argenziano, G., Zalaudek, I., Soyer, H. P., Sera, F. et al. Dermatoscopy of basal cell carcinoma: morphologic variability of global and local features and accuracy of diagnosis. *J. Am. Acad. Dermatol.* 2010;62:67-75.

[30] Rubin, A. I., Chen, E. H., Ratner, D., Basal-Cell Carcinoma. *N. Engl. J. Med.* 2005; 353:2262-69.

[31] Jimenez, F. J., Burchette, J. L., Grichnik, J. M., Hitchcock, M. G. Ber-EP4 immunoreactivity in normal skin and cutaneous neoplasms. *Modern Pathology.* 1995;8:854-58.

[32] Barrett, T. L., Smith, K. J., Hodge, J. J., Butler, R., Hall, F. W., Skelton, H. G. Immunohistochemical nuclear staining for p53, PCNA, and Ki-67 in different histologic variants of basal cell carcinoma. *J. Am. Acad. Dermatol.* 1997;37:430-37.

[33] Poniecka, A. W., Alexis, J. B. An immunohistochemical study of basal cell carcinoma and trichoepithelioma. *Am. J. Dermatopathol.* 1999;21: 332-36.

[34] Amici, J. M., Beylot-Barry, M. [Locally advanced basal-cell carcinoma: Combined alternative treatments beyond surgery]. *Ann. Chir. Plast. Esthet.* 2015;60:321-25.

[35] Burch, M. B., Chung, T. K., Rosenthal, E. L., Schmalbach, C. E. Multimodality management of high-risk head and neck basal cell carcinoma requiring free-flap reconstruction. *Otolaryngol. Head Neck Surg.* 2015;152:868-73.

[36] Roozeboom, M. H., van Kleef, L., Arits, A. H., Mosterd, K., Winnepenninckx, V. J., van Marion, A. M. et al. Tumor thickness and adnexal extension of superficial basal cell carcinoma (sBCC) as determinants of treatment failure for methylaminolevulinate (MAL)-photodynamic therapy (PDT), imiquimod, and 5-fluorouracil (FU). *J. Am. Acad. Dermatol.* 2015;73:93-98.

[37] Nguyen, B. T., Gan, S. D., Konnikov, N., Liang, C. A. Treatment of superficial basal cell carcinoma and squamous cell carcinoma in situ on the trunk and extremities with ablative fractional laser-assisted delivery of topical fluorouracil. *J. Am. Acad. Dermatol.* 2015;72:558-60.

[38] Sollena, P., Del Regno, L., Fargnoli, M. C., Peris, K. Topical and systemic medical treatments of basal cell carcinoma. *G. Ital. Dermatol. Venereol*. 2015;150:429-34.

[39] Sekulic, A., Migden, M. R., Lewis, K., Hainsworth, J. D., Solomon, J. A., Yoo, S. et al. Pivotal ERIVANCE basal cell carcinoma (BCC) study: 12-month update of efficacy and safety of vismodegib in advanced BCC. *J. Am. Acad. Dermatol*. 2015;72:1021-26.e8.

[40] Clausen, O. P., Beigi, M., Bolund, L., Kølvraa, S., Gjersvik, P. J., Mørk, G., de Angelis, P. M. Keratoacanthomas frequently show chromosomal aberrations as assessed by comparative genomic hybridization. *J. Invest. Dermatol*. 2002;119:1367-72.

[41] Clausen, O. P., Aass, H. C., Beigi, M., Purdie, K. J., Proby, C. M., Brown, V. L. et al. Are keratoacanthomas variants of squamous cell carcinomas? A comparison of chromosomal aberrations by comparative genomic hybridization. *J. Invest. Dermatol*. 2006; 126: 2308-15.

[42] Li, J., Wang, K., Gao, F., Jensen, T. D., Li, S. T., DeAngelis, P. M. et al. Array comparative genomic hybridization of keratoacanthomas and squamous cell carcinomas: different patterns of genetic aberrations suggest two distinct entities. *J. Invest. Dermatol*. 2012; 132: 2060-66.

[43] Calcaianu, N., Popescu, S. A., Diveica, D., Lascar, I. Surgical attitude in premalignant lesions and malignant tumors of the lower lip. *J. Med. Life*. 2015;8:109-11.

[44] Ochsenius, G., Ormeño, A., Godoy, L., Rojas, R. [A retrospective study of 232 cases of lip cancer and pre cancer in Chilean patients. Clinical-histological correlation]. *Rev. Med. Chil*. 2003;131:60-66.

[45] Khan, S. U., O'Connor, T. E., Keogh, I. J. A Series of Oral Lesions Presenting to an Otolaryngology Department. *Ir. Med. J*. 2015;108:177-79.

[46] Dejaco, D., Hauser, U., Zelger, B., Riechelmann, H. [Actinic Keratosis]. *Laryngorhinootologie*. 2015;94:467-81.

[47] Majores, M., Bierhoff, E. [Actinic keratosis, Bowen's disease, keratoacanthoma and squamous cell carcinoma of the skin]. *Pathologe*. 2015;36:16-29.

[48] Seidenberg, A. B., Mahalingam-Dhingra, A., Weinstock, M. A., Sinclair, C., Geller, A. C. Youth indoor tanning and skin *Am. J. Prev. Med*. 2015;48:188-94.

[49] Chockalingam, R., Downing, C., Tyring, S. K. Cutaneous squamous cell *J. Clin. Med*. 2015;4:1229-39.

[50] Stratigos, A., Garbe, C., Lebbe, C., Malvehy, J., Del Marmol, V., Pehamberger, H. et al. Diagnosis and treatment of invasive squamous cell carcinoma of the skin: European consensus-based interdisciplinary guideline. *Eur. J. Cancer.* 2015 Jul. 25.pii: S0959-8049(15)00625-5. doi: 10.1016/j.ejca.2015.06.110.

[51] Farrahi, F., Egbert, B. M., Swetter, S. M. Histologic similarities between lentigomaligna and dysplastic nevus: importance of clinicopathologic distinction. *J. Cutan. Pathol.* 2005;32:405-2. Erratum in: *J. Cutan. Pathol.* 2005;32:521.

[52] Rosendahl, C. O., Grant-Kels, J. M., Que, S. K. Dysplastic nevus: Fact and fiction. *J. Am. Acad. Dermatol.* 2015. pii: S0190-9622(15)01598-04.

[53] Crowson, A. N., Magro, C. M., Sanchez-Carpintero, I., Mihm, M. C. Jr. The precursors of malignant melanoma. *Recent Results Cancer Res.* 2002;160:75-84.

[54] Crowson, A. N., Magro, C. M., Mihm, M. C. Jr. Malignant melanoma with prominent pigment synthesis: "animal type" melanoma--a clinical and histological study of six cases with a consideration of other melanocytic neoplasms with prominent pigment synthesis. *Hum. Pathol.* 1999;30:543-50.

[55] Magro, C. M., Crowson, A. N., Mihm, M. C. Unusual variants of malignant melanoma. *Mod. Pathol.* 2006;19 Suppl. 2:S41-70.

[56] Abbasi, N. R., Yancovitz, M., Gutkowicz-Krusin, D., Panageas, K. S., Mihm, M. C., Googe, P., King, R., Prieto, V., Osman, I., Friedman, R. J., Rigel, D. S., Kopf, A. W., Polsky, D. Utility of lesion diameter in the clinical diagnosis of cutaneous melanoma. *Arch. Dermatol.* 2008;144: 469-74.

[57] Kucher, C., Zhang, P. J., Acs, G., Roberts, S., Xu, X. Can Melan-A replace S-100 and HMB-45 in the evaluation of sentinel lymph nodes from patients with malignant melanoma? *Appl. Immunohistochem. Mol. Morphol.* 2006;14:324-27.

[58] Yu, C. H., Chen, H. H., Liu, C. M., Jeng, Y. M., Wang, J. T., Wang, Y. P., Liu, B. Y., Sun, A., Chiang, C. P. HMB-45 may be a more sensitive maker than S-100 or Melan-A for immunohistochemical diagnosis of primary oral and nasal mucosal melanomas. *J. Oral Pathol. Med.* 2005; 34:540-45.

[59] Bhawan, J. Mel-5: a novel antibody for differential diagnosis of epidermal pigmented lesions of the skin in paraffin-embedded sections. *Melanoma Res.* 1997;7:43-48.

[60] Aung, P. P., Sarlomo-Rikala, M., Lasota, J., Lai, J. P., Wang, Z. F., Miettinen, M. KBA62 and PNL2: 2 new melanoma markers-immunohistochemical analysis of 1563 tumors including metastatic, desmoplastic, and mucosal melanomas and their mimics. *Am. J. Surg. Pathol.* 2012;36:265-72.

[61] van Beek, E. J., Balm, A. J., Nieweg, O. E., Hamming-Vrieze, O., Lohuis, P. J., C. Klop, W. M. Treatment of Regional Metastatic Melanoma of Unknown Primary Origin. *Cancers* (Basel). 2015;7:1543-53.

[62] Anisimovvv, semiletovayv, gaftongi, lemekhov vg, myasnyankin my, gaftonig. [comparative evaluation of surgical approaches to treatment of patients with skin melanoma]. *Vopr. Onkol.* 2015;61:387-92.

[63] Bayless, H., Schneider, S. Nivolumab: Immunotherapy in Malignant Melanoma. *Clin. J. Oncol. Nurs.* 2015;19:430-32.

[64] Czajkowski, R., Placek, W., Drewa, G., Czajkowska, A., Uchańska, G. FAMMM syndrome: pathogenesis and management. *Dermatol. Surg.* 2004;30(2 Pt 2):291-96.

[65] Tchernev, G., Ananiev, J., Cardoso, J. C., Chokoeva, A. A., Philipov, S., Penev, P. K. et al. Multiple primary cutaneous melanomas in patients with FAMMM syndrome and sporadic atypical mole syndrome (AMS): what's worse? *Wien. Med. Wochenschr.* 2014;164:302-07.

[66] Takeda, K., Yasumoto, K., Takada, R., Takada, S., Watanabe, K., Udono, T. et al. S.Induction of melanocyte-specific microphthalmia-associated transcription factor by Wnt-3a. *J. Biol. Chem.* 2000;12: 14013-16.

[67] Ehsani, L., Cohen, C., Fisher, K. E., Siddiqui, M. T. BRAF mutations in metastatic malignant melanoma: comparison of molecular analysis and immunohistochemical expression. *Appl. Immunohistochem. Mol. Morphol.* 2014;22:648-51.

[68] Mascarenhas, J. B., Littlejohn, E. L., Wolsky, R. J., Young, K. P., Nelson, M., Salgia, R. et al. DPAX3 and SOX10 activate MET receptor expression in melanoma. *Pigment Cell Melanoma Res.* 2010;23:225-27.

[69] Nonaka, D., Chiriboga, L., Rubin, B. P. Sox10: a pan-schwannian and melanocytic marker. *Am. J. Surg. Pathol.* 2008;32:1291-98.

[70] Wolf, I. H., Kodama, K., Cerroni, L., Kerl, H. Nature of inflammatory infiltrate in superficial cutaneous malignancies during topical imiquimod treatment. *Am. J. Dermatopathol.* 2007;29:237-41.

[71] Adams, S., O'Neill, D. W., Nonaka, D., Hardin, E., Chiriboga, L., Siu, K. et al. Immunization of malignant melanoma patients with full-length

NY-ESO-1 protein using TLR7 agonist imiquimod as vaccine adjuvant. *J. Immunol.* 2008;1:776-84.

[72] http://www.cancer.org/acs/groups/cid/documents/webcontent/002550-pdf.pdf.

[73] Makkouk, A., Joshi, V. B., Wongrakpanich, A., Lemke, C. D., Gross, B. P., Salem, A. K. et al. Biodegradable microparticles loaded with doxorubicin and CpG ODN for in situ immunization against cancer. *AAPS J.* 2015;17:184-93.

[74] Sousa, S. F., Gomez, R. S., Diniz, M. G., Bernardes, V. F., Soares, F. F., Brito, J. A. et al. Defects of the Carney complex gene (PRKAR1A) in odontogenic tumors *Endocr. Relat. Cancer.* 2015;3:399-408.

[75] Fukuoka, H., Takahashi, Y. The role of genetic and epigenetic changes in pituitary tumorigenesis *Neurol. Med. Chir.* (Tokyo). 2014;54:943-57.

[76] Torres-Mora, J., Dry, S., Li, X., Binder, S., Amin, M., Folpe, A. L. Malignant melanoticschwannian tumor: a clinicopathologic, immunohistochemical, and gene expression profiling study of 40 cases, with a proposal for the reclassification of "melanoticschwannoma." *Am. J. Surg. Pathol.* 2014;38:94-05.

[77] Shanmugam, S., Ghosh, M., Niamathullah, S., Ghosh, S. Psammomatous melanotic schwannoma as a component of Carney complex. *Indian J. Pathol. Microbiol.* 2015;58:368-70.

[78] Plotkin, S. R., Albers, A. C., Babovic-Vuksanovic, D., Blakeley, J. O., Breakefield, X. O., Dunn, C. M. et al. Update from the 2013 International Neurofibromatosis Conference. *Am. J. Med. Genet. A.* 2014;164A:2969-78.

[79] Rodrigues, L. O., Batista, P. B., Goloni-Bertollo, E. M., de Souza-Costa, D., Eliam, L., Eliam, M., Cunha, K. S. et al. Neurofibromatoses: part 1 - diagnosis and differential diagnosis. *Arq. Neuropsiquiatr.* 2014;72:241-50.

[80] Merker, V. L., Bredella, M. A., Cai, W., Kassarjian, A., Harris, G. J., Muzikansky, A. et al. Relationship between whole-body tumor burden, clinical phenotype, and quality of life in patients with neurofibromatosis. *Am. J. Med. Genet. A.* 2014;164A:1431-37.

[81] Korf, B. R. The phakomatoses. *Clin. Dermatol.* 2005;23:78-84.

[82] Fletcher, C. D. Solitary circumscribed neuroma of the skin (so-called palisaded, encapsulated neuroma). A clinicopathologic and immunohistochemical study. *Am. J. Surg. Pathol.* 1989;13:574-80.

[83] Guillet, G., Gauthier, Y., Tamisier, J. M., Geniaux, M., Leroy, J. P., Texier, L. et al. Linear cutaneous neuromas (dermatoneurieenstries): a

limited phakomatosis with striated pigmentation corresponding to cutaneous hyperneury (featuring multiple endocrine neoplasia syndrome?). *J. Cutan. Pathol.* 1987;14:43-48.
[84] Bhatt, T. A., Mimesh, S. Cutaneous hyperneury: a new entity or an atypical cutaneous manifestation of MEN 2B? *Skinmed.* 2015;13:145-46.
[85] McLaughlin, C. T., Kaffenberger, B. H., Gru, A. A. A hybrid tumor with schwannoma-perineurioma-neurofibroma morphology. *J. Cutan. Pathol.* 2015 Jul. 3.doi: 10.1111/cup.12544.
[86] Truchot, F., Grézard, P., Wolf, F., Balme, B., Perrot, H. Multiple idiopathic mucocutaneous neuromas: a new entity? *Br. J. Dermatol.* 2001;145:826-29.
[87] Kuruvila, S., Ramadan, F. A. Bednar tumor. *Saudi Med. J.* 2004;25: 2016-17.
[88] Zhang, J., Zhang, R. S., Wei, X., Shi, Q. L., Zhou, X. J., Ma, J. [Pigmented dermatofibrosarcoma protuberance: a clinicopathologic analysis of 7 cases]. *Zhonghua Bing Li Xue Za Zhi.* 2013;42:810-14.
[89] Aziz, R., Jamil, A. Dermatofibrosarcoma: a rare neoplasm of skin. *BMJ Case Rep.* 2012; 21;2012. pii: bcr2012007300.
[90] Tardío, J. C., Pinedo, F., Aramburu, J. A., Suárez-Massa, D., Pampín, A., Requena, L., Santonja, C. Pleomorphic dermal sarcoma: a more aggressive neoplasm than previously estimated. *J. Cutan. Pathol.* 2015 Aug. 12.doi: 10.1111/cup.12603.

In: Inflammatory Markers, Oncogenes … ISBN: 978-1-63484-303-4
Editor: Ana Maria Abreu Velez

Chapter 2

Vimentin, Bromodeoxyuridine and Topoisomerase II A Expression in a Mildly Dysplastic Compound Nevus

Ana Maria Abreu Velez[1,*], MD, PhD, Carlos Andres Valencia-Yepes[2], MSc and Michael S. Howard[1], MD

[1]Georgia Dermatopathology Associates, Atlanta, Georgia, US
[2]Neuroscience Group, University of Antioquia, Medellin, Colombia, South America

Abstract

Context: Dysplastic nevi are atypical, yet benign melanocytic nevi. Dysplastic nevi may present some clinical features of melanoma; histologically, hallmark features of dysplastic nevi include architectural disorder and cytologic atypia of melanocytes. The medical literature indicates that 2 to 8 percent of Caucasian populations have dysplastic nevi. Inheritance seems to play a part in DN development. We present a case of a DN, with positive immunohistochemistry staining for selected cell cycle markers. *Case report:* A 45 male presented to the dermatologist

* Corresponding author: Ana Maria Abreu Velez, MD, PhD, Georgia Dermatopathology Associates, 1534 North Decatur Road., NE; Suite 206; Atlanta, Georgia 30307-1000 US, Telephone: (404) 371-0077, Toll Free: (877) 371-0027, Fax: (404) 371-1900, E-mail: abreuvelez@yahoo.com.

for evaluation of a flat, hyperpigmented macule on his back. A skin biopsy was taken for hematoxylin and eosin (H&E) review and for immunohistochemistry (IHC) staining. The IHC staining for topoisomerase IIα and bromodeoxyuridine was positive on several cells located along the basement membrane zone (BMZ) of the epidermis, and also on some dermal, perivascular inflammatory cells subjacent to the DN. HMB-45 and tyrosinase stains were positive in local nested areas along the BMZ. S-100 and CD68 were positive along the BMZ where the dysplastic melanocytes were present, and also under the DN in the inflammatory infiltrate. Utilizing vimentin IHC staining, we discovered that some type of signaling occurs around the dysplastic nevus cells in the DN. We suggest further study of how cell cycle regulators seem to work "in block" not only within dysplastic nevi, but also surrounding them. Moreover, the immunologic microenvironment of dysplastic nevi and their surrounding cells is poorly understood.

Keywords: dysplastic nevus (DN), vimentin, bromodeoxyuridine, topoisomerase IIα

Abbreviations

H&E	Hematoxylin and eosin
IHC	immunohistochemistry
DAB	3,3-diaminobenzidine
DN	dysplastic nevus
BMZ	basement membrane zone
Topo	topoisomerase IIα

Introduction

Dysplastic nevi (also called "atypical nevi") are sporadic, acquired melanocytic nevi that may present some clinical features of melanoma. Severely dysplastic nevi are more closely associated with development of melanoma than lesser grades of atypia, including mild and moderately dysplastic nevi.

People who have dysplastic nevi are at higher risk of developing single or multiple melanomas [1-4]. It is also believed that the greater the number of dysplastic nevi, the greater the risk; those who have 10 or more have 12 times the danger of developing melanoma relative to the general population. Moreover, dysplastic nevi are found more often in melanoma patients than in the general population [1-4]. Those who have dysplastic nevi in addition to a family history of melanoma have a very high risk of developing melanoma. Histologically, dysplastic nevi display architectural abnormalities and cytological atypia [1-4].

People with dysplastic nevi and a family history of dysplastic nevi and melanoma tend to develop melanoma at an earlier age than melanoma patients who do not have such a family history. Individuals who have dysplastic nevi but no family history of DN or melanoma may also develop melanoma at a relatively early age, but less often. Sometimes it is difficult to clinically distinguish between dysplastic nevi, versus early melanomas beginning within a dysplastic nevus.

Materials and Methods

A skin biopsy for hematoxylin and eosin (H&E) review and for immunohistochemistry (IHC) staining were processed as previously described [5-7].

Immunohistochemistry (IHC)

We performed IHC utilizing multiple monoclonal and polyclonal antibodies from Dako (Carpinteria, California, US) as previously described [7-9]. We utilized 1) mouse anti-human bromodeoxyuridine, clone Bu20a; 2) CD68, clone EBM11; 3) melanosome, clone HMB-45, and 4) topoisomerase IIα (Topo), clone Ki-S1.

We also used a polyclonal rabbit anti-human S-100 antibody (reacts strongly with human S100B, and weakly or very weakly with S100A1 and S100A6, respectively). We also use the antibody tyrosinase clone T311 and Vimentin from Leica. Positive and negative controls were consistently performed.

RESULTS

H&E Staining

Our H&E staining showed lesional melanocytes with epidermal junctional extension beyond the dermal component, some bridging of rete ridges, and focal dermal fibrosis. Some lesional melanocytic cytological atypia was seen including large nuclear size, prominence of nucleoli, hyperchromasia and variation in nuclear staining. There was considerable variability in nuclear shape. The cytoplasm was occasionally collapsed to form a clear space, or halo, around the cell. The diagnosis of a mildly dysplastic compound nevus was made (Figure 1). A superficial, perivascular dermal inflammatory infiltrate was also noted in the subjacent dermis below the DN.

IHC Staining

HMB-45 and tyrosinase were positive along the basement membrane zone (BMZ), with additional nests of positive staining within the dermis. Staining for topoisomerase IIα and bromodeoxyuridine was positive on several lesional cells located along the basement membrane zone (BMZ) of the epidermis, and also on some dermal inflammatory cells under the DN. S-100 and CD68 were positive along the BMZ on or near the dysplastic melanocytes, and also under the DN in the subjacent dermis (Figure 1). Vimentin was also positive along the BMZ around the DN, and also under the DN in the subjacent dermis.

DISCUSSION

Nevi with architectural disorder and cytologic atypia of melanocytes are termed "dysplastic nevi." They have variable degrees of histologic abnormalities, which can be classified on a spectrum of atypia as "mild," "moderate" or "severe." Grading encompasses both architectural and cytological features, which often correlate with each other. Architectural criteria include asymmetry, bridging of epidermal rete ridges by nevus cell nests, and lamellar fibroplasia of lesional dermal collagen [1-4].

On H&E review, we established the diagnosis of a mildly dysplastic compound nevus.

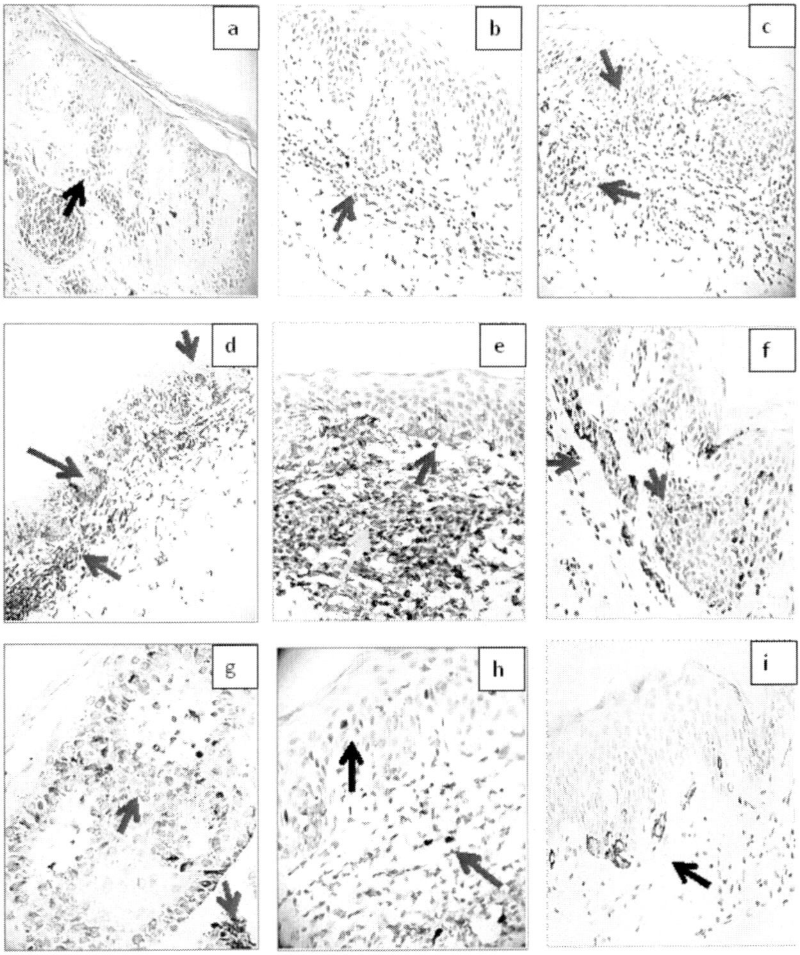

Figure 1. a. H&E image of the dysplastic nevus. A melanocytic cell nest is highlighted at an epidermal rete ridge tip (black arrow) (200X). b. IHC staining with CD68, showing positive staining among inflammatory cells under the DN (brown staining; red arrow). c. IHC staining with S-100, showing positive melanocytic cell nest staining along the BMZ. Positive staining is also noted in the dermal perivascular inflammatory infiltrate below the DN (brown staining; red arrows). d and e. Positive IHC staining with vimentin around DN nests along the BMZ (brown staining; red arrows), and also in the subjacent dermis (brown staining; blue and yellow arrows). f and g. Positive IHC staining with bromodeoxyuridine in the DN, and subjacent to the lesion (brown staining; red arrows). h. Positive IHC staining with topoisomerase along the BMZ (brown staining; black arrow), and also on subjacent dermal inflammatory cells (brown staining; red arrow). i. Positive IHC staining for HMB-45 along the BMZ, in DN junctional cell nests (brown staining; black arrow).

We then observed positive IHC staining for melanocytic markers such tyrosinase and HMB-45 on nevus melanocytes. In these same areas, we noted positive IHC staining for cell cycle markers; these markers included topoisomerase IIα enzymes, which control DNA topology in cell replication by cleaving, cutting and rejoining DNA strands and passing other DNA strands through the transient gaps. The topoisomerase IIα enzyme isoform is a 170 kDa nuclear protein that is only expressed in proliferating cells. We also noted positive staining in these areas for bromodeoxyuridine. The bromodeoxyuridine marker binds to replicating cells which have incorporated bromodeoxyuridine into their DNA during the S-phase of the cell cycle.

We also noted that IHC staining for S-100 and CD68 was positive in the lesional area, possibly highlighting Langerhans and non-Langerhans antigen presenting cells around the DN.

We noted interesting findings in our positive IHC staining for vimentin. Vimentin is a 57 kDa intermediate filament protein, and a component of the cytoskeleton of vertebrate cells; it is characteristically found in cells of mesenchymal origin. We noted vimentin staining along the BMZ around DN nests, and within the dermis subjacent to the DN.

In the medical literature, little attention has focused on the immunologic environment around dysplastic nevi. In our vimentin staining, we note a suggestion of immune system mesenchymal cell movement and/or response around DN nests, and beyond the immediate area of the DN. Other authors have recently studied how cancer cells metastasize through the blood, via lymphatics, along nerves or by other modalities [9]. They found that cells in each microanatomic area of the primary tumor exhibited either fast or slow locomotion [9]. To understand how the tumor microenvironment thus influences tumor cell locomotion, invasion, migration and immune response resistance, many studies are warranted. As shown in our case, the immunologic microenvironment of dysplastic nevi warrants further study; these studies would increase our understanding of the neoplastic process, and confirm any potential markers for malignant transformation.

ACKNOWLEDGMENTS

Jonathan S. Jones, HT(ASCP) at Georgia Dermatopathology Associates provided excellent technical assistance.

Conflicts of interest

None.

Funding

Georgia Dermatopathology Associates, Atlanta, Georgia, US.

REFERENCES

[1] Clark, W. H. Jr, Reimer, R. R., Greene, M., Ainsworth, A. M., Mastrangelo, M. J. Origin of familial malignant melanomas from heritable melanocytic lesions. "The B-K mole syndrome." *Arch. Dermatol.* 1978;114:732-8.

[2] Clark, W. H. Jr. The dysplastic nevus syndrome. *Arch. Dermatol.* 1988; 124:1207-10.

[3] Clark, W. H. Jr, Elder, D. E., Guerry, D. I. V., Epstein, M. N., Greene, M. H., Van Horn, M. A study of tumor progression: the precursor lesions of superficial spreading and nodular melanoma. *Hum. Pathol.* 1984;15:1147-55.

[4] Elder, D. E., Goldman, L. I., Goldman, S. C., Greene, M. H., Clark, W. H. Jr. Dysplastic nevus syndrome: a phenotypic association of sporadic cutaneous melanoma. *Cancer* 1980;46:1787-94.

[5] Abreu Velez, A. M., Howard, M. S. Immune reactivity in psoriatic Munro-Saboureau microabscesses, stratum corneum and blood vessels. *North Am. J. Med. Sci.* 2012;4: 257-85.

[6] Abreu Velez, A. M., Howard, M. S., Gao, W., Grossniklaus, H. E., Zhe, J., Arias, L. F., Dudley, S. C., Smoller, B. R. Varicella-zoster virus (VZV), and alpha 1 antitrypsin: a fatal outcome in a patient affected by endemic pemphigus. *Int. J. Dermatol.* 2012;51:809-16.

[7] Abreu Velez, A. M., Howard, M. S. Collagen IV in normal skin and in pathologic processes. *North Am. J. Med. Sci.* 2012; 4:1-8.

[8] Arumi-Uria, M., McNutt, N. S., Finnerty, B. Grading of Atypia in Nevi: Correlation with Melanoma Risk. *Mod. Pathol.* 2003;16:764-71.

[9] Gligorijevic, B., Bergman, A., Condeelis, J. Multiparametric Classification Links Tumor Microenvironments with Tumor Cell Phenotype. *PLoS Biol.* 2014;12(11): e1001995.

In: Inflammatory Markers, Oncogenes … ISBN: 978-1-63484-303-4
Editor: Ana Maria Abreu Velez

Chapter 3

A BASAL CELL CARCINOMA WITH SEBACEOUS AND SQUAMOUS DIFFERENTIATION, WITH EXPRESSION OF PROLIFERATING CELL NUCLEAR ANTIGEN, P27^{KIP1} AND VIMENTIN

Ana Maria Abreu Velez[1,*], MD, PhD,
DA Vásquez-Hincapié[2], MD
and Michael S. Howard[1], MD
[1]Georgia Dermatopathology Associates, Atlanta, GA, US
[2]Pecet, University of Antioquia, Medellin, Colombia

ABSTRACT

Context: Some authors have used sebaceous epithelioma or sebaceoma as synonyms for basal cell carcinoma (BCC) with sebaceous differentiation; these lesions may be difficult to diagnose, and little is known about their cell cycle regulator marker expression.

[*] Corresponding author: Ana Maria Abreu Velez, MD, PhD, Georgia Dermatopathology Associates, 1534 North Decatur Road., NE; Suite 206; Atlanta, Georgia 30307-1000 USA. E-mail: abreuvelez@yahoo.com, Tel.: (404) 371-0077, Toll Free: (877) 371-0027, Fax: (404) 371-1900.

Case Report: A 74 year old female noted a nodule on her back, with some inflammation. She consulted her dermatologist.

Materials and Methods. A skin biopsy for hematoxylin and eosin (H&E) and for immunohistochemistry (IHC) staining was taken.

Results: H&E staining showed a neoplastic process largely composed of basaloid keratinocytes, and displaying focal squamous and sebaceous differentiation within the tumor. Some peripheral palisaded areas of basaloid keratinocytes were appreciated. By IHC, the epithelial cell antigen clone AE1/AE3was positive in squamous differentiated areas of the tumor. Human epithelial antigen (Ber-EP4) was also focally positive, and proliferating cell nuclear antigen (PCNA) was very positive in basaloid areas of the tumor. $P27^{Kip1}$ was positive in the well differentiated, sebaceous areas of the tumor. Vimentin was positive in tumor stromal areas, between the tumor cells. We found positiveCDX2 stain on a few edges of the tumor, in squamous differentiated areas. The host immune response to the tumor was scant.

Conclusion: We document a mixed differentiation tumor, and document significant PCNA positivity. In addition, vimentin proved to be an excellent marker for highlighting tumor lobules.

Keywords: basal cell carcinoma with sebaceous and squamous differentiation, cell cycle regulators, human epithelial antigen, (Ber-EP4), proliferating cell nuclear antigen (PCNA), vimentin, $p27^{Kip1}$

Abbreviations

H&E	Hematoxylin and eosin
IHC	immunohistochemistry
AE1/AE3	pancytokeratin
DAB	3,3-diaminobenzidine
LAT	linker for activation of T cells
BCL-2	B-celllymphoma 2 gene
PCNA	proliferating cell nuclear antigen
Ber-EP4	human epithelial antigen

Introduction

Basal cell carcinoma (BCC) is one of the most common forms of human cancer. Increased expression of p53 has been found in the majority of BCCs.

Most well differentiated BCCs label with human epithelial antigen, clone Ber-EP4 [1-6]. Thus, Ber-EP4 antigen aids in the diagnosis of basal cell, squamous cell and basosquamous carcinomas of the skin [1-6]. Some cutaneous basaloid keratinocytic neoplasms also display sebaceous differentiation. Ultraviolet (UV) radiation-induced signature mutations seem to be present in only about 50% of cases of BCCs. Increased nuclear staining with an immunohistochemical marker of proliferation and apoptosis has been correlated with aggressive behavior in BCCs. A basal cell carcinoma with sebaceous differentiation represents a lesion of borderline malignancy [7].

Case Report

A 74 year old female presented with a nodule on her back with some inflammation. She consulted her dermatologist, and a skin biopsy for hematoxylin and eosin (H&E) and for immunohistochemistry (IHC) stains was taken. Following the diagnosis, a surgical removal of the lesion was performed.

Materials and Methods

Immunohistochemistry (IHC)

We performed IHC utilizing multiple monoclonal and polyclonal antibodies from Dako (Carpinteria, California, USA) as previously described [7-9]. We utilized mouse anti-humanbromodeoxyuridine, clone Bu20a; human epithelial antigen, clone Ber-EP4; $p27^{Kip1}$, clone SX53G8; Cyclin D1, clone EP12; p53; BRCA-1; proliferating cell nuclear antigen (PCNA), clone PC10; pancytokeratin, clone AE1/AE3; anti-human-BRCA-1, clone GLK-2; Cytokeratin 20; chromogranin A, clone DAK-A3; Alpha 1 antitrypsin, ZAP-70;LAT protein, clone LAT-1; B-celllymphoma 2 gene (BCL-2) oncoprotein, clone 124; BCL-6; BCL-10;CDX2, clone DAK-CDX2; tissue inhibitor of metalloproteinase (TIMP-1) and matrix-metalloproteinase 9 (MMP9) clone A0150.

Single Color Immunohistochemistry

For our IHC testing, we utilized a dual endogenous peroxidase blockage, with the addition of a Dako Envision dual link (to assist in chromogen attachment). We then applied the chromogen 3,3-diaminobenzidine (DAB), and counterstained with hematoxylin. The samples were run in a Dako Autostainer Universal Staining System. Positive and negative controls were consistently performed. The staining was performed as previously described [7-9].

RESULTS

Microscopic Description

H and E Staining

Examination of the tissue sections demonstrates a neoplasm, originating from the epidermis and comprised of focal aggregates of atypical basaloid keratinocytes admixed with a minority population of sebocytes. Focal keratinized areas and stroma were also present within the tumor (Figure 1). The tumor was well circumscribed, and extended into the dermis. The basaloid keratinocytes displayed round, regular nuclei with fine, dispersed chromatin; minimal amounts of basophilic cytoplasm are present within these cells. Palisading of peripheral nuclei within the tumor aggregates was also observed.

IHC Stains

The positive controls stained appropriately. Ber-EP4 was focally positive, present in basaloid keratinocytic areas of the tumor. PancytokeratinAE1/AE3 was positive in areas of squamous differentiation (Figure 1). Chromogranin A, bromodeoxyuridine, Cytokeratin 20, BRCA-1, p53, cyclin D1, ZAP70, LAT, alpha 1 antitrypsin, metalloproteinase 9, BCL-2, BCL-6, BCL-10 and tissue inhibitor of metalloproteinase 1(TIMP-1) were negative. Vimentin was positive in stromal areas of the tumor (Figure 1). CDX2 was positive in some of the keratinized, squamous areas of the tumor. $P27^{Kip1}$ was positive exclusively in well differentiated, sebaceous areas of the tumor. PCNA was very positive, throughout basaloid areas of the tumor. Vimentin was positive in the stromal areas between the lobules of the tumor (Figure 1).

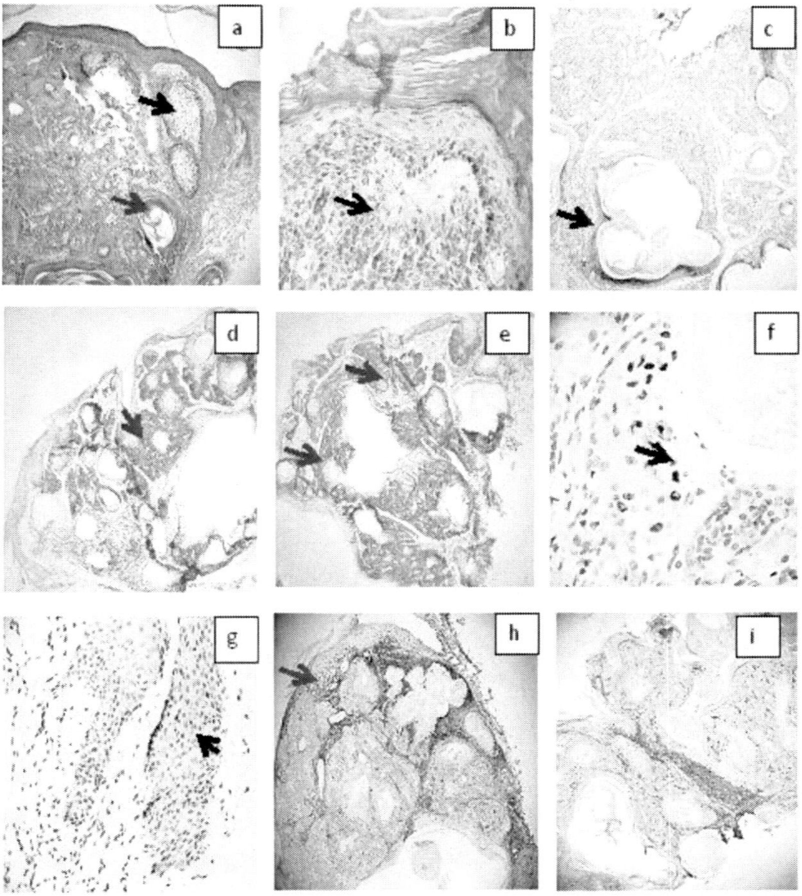

Figure 1. a and b. Shows H&E staining of the tumor at 100 and 200X magnifications, respectively. In a, the red arrow indicates tumoral squamous differentiation, and in b the black arrow highlights a nearby sebaceous gland. c. IHC staining, showing positive staining with Cytokeratin AE1/AE3 in keratinized areas of the tumor (brown staining; black arrow). d and e. IHC staining using PCNA, showing diffusely positive staining in basaloid areas of the tumor (brown staining; red arrows). f. IHC positive staining for $p27^{Kip1}$, highlighting sebaceous differentiation within the tumor (brown staining; black arrow). g. IHC positive staining at the edge of the tumor with CDX2 (brown staining; black arrow). Finally, in h and i, IHC positive staining in the stromal area of the tumor with vimentin (brown staining; red arrow).

DISCUSSION

Human epithelial antigen IHC staining of basal cell carcinomas is well documented. In this case, we observed focal, tumoral Ber-EP4 staining. Our Ber-EP4 findings are consistent with our H&E diagnosis of a basal cell carcinoma with sebaceous and squamous differentiation. Interesting aspects of the tumor IHC include diffuse basaloid PCNA staining, and diffuse vimentin stromal staining. We also noted that the immune response to the tumor was scant.

Other authors have also reported IHC PCNA positivity in other skin cancers and skin proliferative disorders using semiquantitative analysis. These authors studied the expression of PCNA in seborrheic keratoses (SKs), actinic keratoses (AKs), Bowen's disease (BD), and squamous cell carcinoma (SCC) [10]. The authors suggested that their observed PCNA expression was related to the degree of cell proliferation [10]. Another group of authors studied PCNA and other markers in BCCs to correlate markers of apoptosis (p53 and BCL-2) and cell proliferation (Ki-67 and PCNA) with histological indicators of tumor severity [11]. The authors specifically studied IHC stains for p53, BCL-2, PCNA, and Ki-67 in superficial, nodular and sclerosing BCCs. The authors did not study BCCs with sebaceous differentiation. They found that BCL-2 expression was significantly increased in clinically aggressive BCCs (morpheaform and nodular types). Of the studied tumors, 66.7% (n = 14) strongly expressed p53 [11]. The authors showed a greater relative expression of Ki-67 in nodular and superficial BCCs, and they found that PCNA displayed strong expression in all BCC types. Our findings in our BCC with sebaceous differentiation are consistent with their findings; specifically, we noted strongly positive PCNA expression in basaloid areas.

Another group of authors studied seven cases of BCC with sebaceous differentiation, using IHC testing for cellular proliferation via proliferating cell nuclear antigen (PCNA) and Ki-67. They suggested that semi-quantitative grading of PCNA and Ki-67 staining could be useful in differentiating BCC from basal cell carcinoma with sebaceous differentiation (BCSD) [12]. We have recently reviewed cell cycle regulatory checkpoints and the skin, and their relevance is illustrated in our PCNA findings [13].

In addition to PCNA, we found positiveCDX2 staining on some edges of the tumor. CDX2 is a human gene homologous to the Drosophila caudal-type homeobox gene. CDX-2 encodes a transcription factor involved in proliferation and differentiation of intestinal epithelial cells, and is not expressed in normal skin. However, CDX-2 expression has been documented in metastatic melanoma and extramammary Paget's disease [14]. We do not know the significance of our CDX-2 staining. We also noted vimentin positivity in stromal areas of our tumor, as well as $p27^{Kip1}$ staining in sebaceous areas. Thus, these markers may be helpful in confirming a diagnosis in similar tumors.

The most challenging area in recommending treatment for our tumor concerned categorizing this lesion relative to a sebaceoma [15]. Indeed, these tumors represent a spectrum of clinical and histologic findings, and their exact classification warrants larger, consolidated studies with multiple IHC markers.

ACKNOWLEDGMENT

Jonathan S. Jones, HT(ASCP) at Georgia Dermatopathology Associates provided excellent technical assistance.

Conflicts of Interest

None.

Funding

Georgia Dermatopathology Associates, Atlanta, Georgia, US.

REFERENCES

[1] Bahar Dasgeb B., Mohammadi T. M., Mehregan D. R. Use of Ber-EP4 and Epithelial Specific Antigen to Differentiate Clinical Simulators of Basal Cell Carcinoma. *Biomark Cancer*. 2013; 5: 7-11.

[2] Tellechea O., Reis J. P., Domingues J. C., Baptista A. P. Monoclonal antibody Ber EP4 distinguishes basal-cell carcinoma from squamous-cell carcinoma of the skin. *Am J Dermatopathol*. 1993; 15: 452-55.

[3] Jimenez F. J., Burchette J. L. Jr., Grichnik J. M., Hitchcock M. G. Ber-EP4 immunoreactivity in normal skin and cutaneous neoplasms. *Mod Pathol*. 1995; 8:854-58.

[4] Swanson P. E., Fitzpatrick M. M., Ritter J. H., Glusac E. J., Wick M. R. Immunohistologic differential diagnosis of basal cell carcinoma, squamous cell carcinoma, and trichoepithelioma in small cutaneous biopsy specimens. *J CutanPathol.* 1998; 25: 153-59.

[5] Beer T. W., Shepherd P., Theaker J. M. Ber EP4 and epithelial membrane antigen aid distinction of basal cell, squamous cell and basosquamous carcinomas of the skin. *Histopathology.* 2000; 37:218-23.

[6] Ansai S., Takeichi H., Arase S., Kawana S., Kimura T. Sebaceous carcinoma: an immunohistochemical reappraisal. *Am J Dermatopathol.* 2011; 33: 579-87.

[7] Abreu Velez A. M., Vásquez-Hincapié D. A., Howard M. S. Vimentin may reflect areas of cutaneous involvement in biopsies from patients with autoimmune skin diseases. *Our Dermatol Online.* 2014; 5: 140-43.

[8] Abreu Velez A. M., Jackson B. L., Velasquez-Cantillo K. L., Benavides-Alvarez A. R., Howard M. S. Merkel cell carcinoma versus metastatic small cell primary bronchogenic carcinoma. *Our Dermatol Online,* 2013; 4: 64-71.

[9] Abreu Velez A. M., Smith J. G. Jr., Howard M. S. Vimentin compartamentalization in discoid lupus. *North Am J Med Sci.* 2010; 2: 106-10.

[10] Tsuji T., Kitajima S., Koashi Y. Expression of proliferating cell nuclear antigen (PCNA) and apoptosis related antigen (LeY) in epithelial skin tumors. *Am J Dermatopathol.* 1998; 20:164-69.

[11] Mateoiu C., Pirici A., Bogdan F. Immunohistochemical nuclear staining for p53 *Rom J Morphol Embryol.* 2011; 52(1 S): 315-19.

[12] Ansai S., Koseki S., Hozumi Y., Kondo S., Aso K. Assessment of cellular proliferation of sebaceous neoplasms by AgNOR counts and immunohistochemical demonstrations of PCNA and Ki-67. *J Dermatol.* 1995; 22: 238-48.

[13] Abreu Velez A. M., Howard M. S. Tumor suppressor genes, cell cycle regulatory checkpoints and the skin. *North Am J Med.* 2015; 7: 176-87.

[14] Lora V., Kanitakis J. CDX2 expression in cutaneous metastatic carcinomas and extramammary Paget's Disease. *Anticancer Res.* 2009; 29: 5033-37.

[15] Misago N., Suse T., Uemura T., Narisawa Y. Basal cell carcinoma with sebaceous differentiation. *Am J Dermatopathol.* 2004; 26: 298-03.

In: Inflammatory Markers, Oncogenes ... ISBN: 978-1-63484-303-4
Editor: Ana Maria Abreu Velez

Chapter 4

A CASE OF AN INFLAMED PRECANCEROUS WART AND IMMUNE RESPONSE WITH FACTOR XIIIA, IGD, CD11C/CD18 AND CD79A

Ana Maria Abreu Velez[1,*], MD, PhD, Billie L. Jackson[2], MD and Michael S. Howard[1], MD
[1]Georgia Dermatopathology Associates, Atlanta, Georgia, US
[2]Dermatologist, Macon, Georgia, US

ABSTRACT

Context: Warts are caused by human papillomaviruses (HPVs); in some cases, warts may contain precancerous histologic features.. Specifically, severe inflammation within warts has been associated with progression to skin cancers. *Case report:* An 82 year old female presented to the dermatologist with an inflamed and itchy plaque, with scaling and a keratotic verrucous surface on her right arm. Materials and methods. A skin biopsy for hematoxylin and eosin (H&E) examination, and for possible immunohistochemistry staining was taken. *Results:* The H&E staining showed epidermal hyperkeratosis, with focal parakeratosis

* Corresponding author: Ana Maria Abreu Velez, MD, PhD, Georgia Dermatopathology Associates, 1534 North Decatur Road., NE; Suite 206; Atlanta, Georgia 30307-1000 USA. E-mail: abreuvelez@yahoo.com, Telephone: (404) 371-0077, Toll Free: (877) 371-0027, Fax: (404) 371-1900.

also present within the stratum corneum. The epidermis displayed papillomatosis, and hypergranulosis. Cells with altered nuclei surrounded by a white halo (koilocytes) were also seen. A focal inflammatory infiltrate was present at the base of the lesion. A diagnosis of an inflamed wart was made. IHC staining showed the basaloid infiltrate to demonstrate positivity with CD11c/CD18, CD79A and IgD. Positive EMA/CD227 and Cytokeratin AE1/AE3 staining was noted in the lesion. *Conclusion.* We found a robust immune response in the wart, without signs of malignant transformation. A wart in an apparently normal individual that suddenly "becomes inflamed" may in fact represent part of a targeted immune response towards the wart viral particles. If these changes consistently fail to occur in patients under immunosuppression due to a transplant, HIV infection or chronic radiotherapy, it is important to test for the integrity of the immune response. Further, if a sudden inflammation of the wart occurs in a senior person, it is important to consider the differential diagnosis of a malignancy.

Keywords: pre-cancer, human papillomavirus (HPV), inflammation, CD11c/CD18, CD15, CD45, pancytokeratin AE1/AE3, epithelial membrane antigen (EMA/CD227), PCNA

Abbreviations

HPVs	Human papillomavirus
H&E	hematoxylin and eosin
IHC	immunohistochemistry
EMA/CD227	epithelial membrane antigen
DAB	3,3-diaminobenzidine

Introduction

Cutaneous infections caused by human papillomavirus (HPVs) are usually recurrent, and are among the most troublesome conditions presenting to dermatologists. Human papillomaviruses (HPVs) are DNA viruses of the papovavirus family, with more than 100 kinds defined [1-4]. Common warts (verrucae vulgaris) are usually caused by HPV serotypes 1, 2, 4 and 7. They are common in children, as well as in the general population. Their impact in human disease is significant because these viruses are among the most common pathogens in cutaneous infectious diseases. In addition, they are causative in a subset of predominantly (but not exclusively) genital squamous cell carcinomas [1-4]. Warts are usually self-limiting, but spontaneous resolution may occur for months to years. Warts are more frequent on the hands, especially on the fingers [1-4] Spontaneous clearance rates are also low (65-78% at 2 years) [1-4]. The fact that they can recur even after complete physical removal makes them annoying both for the patient and the physician. Recalcitrant warts may reflect a localized or systemic cell-mediated immune deficiency to HPV. Warts are often exuberant in patients with Hodgkin's disease, AIDS and those on immunosuppressant's [1-4]. The histologic features of HPV infection are very easy to identify on tissue sections stained with hematoxylin and eosin (H&E).

CASE REPORT

An 82 year old female presented with a plaque with erythema on her right arm. A skin biopsy for hematoxylin and eosin (H&E) histologic staining, and possible immunohistochemical (IHC) staining was taken; processing was performed as previously described [5-11].

MATERIALS AND METHODS

Immunohistochemistry (IHC): We performed IHC utilizing multiple monoclonal and polyclonal antibodies from Dako (Carpinteria, California, USA). We utilized mouse anti-human, IgD, pancytokeratin clone AE1/AE3 and epithelial membrane antigen (EMA/CD227). We also used antibodies to Factor XIIIa, CD11c/CD18 and CD79a from Leica/Novocastra (Buffalo Grove, Illinois USA). Single color immunohistochemistry (IHC): For our IHC testing, we utilized a dual endogenous peroxidase blockage, with the addition of a Dako Envision dual link(to assist in chromogen attachment). We then applied the chromogen 3,3-diaminobenzidine (DAB), and counterstained with hematoxylin. The samples were run in a Dako Autostainer Universal Staining System. Positive and negative controls were consistently performed. Our staining was performed as previously described [5-11]. IHC double staining: These stains were performed utilizing a Leica double staining system. Specifically, for primary staining we utilized a Bond Max platform autostainer with bond polymer refined red detection DS9390, an alkaline phosphatase linker polymer and fast red chromogen (red staining). For our secondary staining, we utilized bond polymer refined detection DS9800, a horseradish peroxidase linker polymer and DAB chromogen (brown staining). Positive and negative controls were consistently performed. Our staining was performed as previously described [5-11].

RESULTS

Microscopic description using H&E stains: Examination of the tissue sections demonstrates an epidermal hyperkeratosis, with focal parakeratosis also present within the stratum corneum. The epidermis also displays papillomatosis, and hypergranulosis [see Figure 1]. Cells with altered nuclei surrounded by a white halo were seen (koilocytes) were seen. A focal inflammatory infiltrate was present at the base of the lesion. Dilated blood vessels were observed within the dermal papillary tips. The lesion appeared free of the specimen borders in the sections examined.

IHC STAINING

Pancytokeratin, clone (AE1/AE3) was positive in the papillomatous areas of the lesion [see Figure 1]. Epithelial membrane antigen (EMA/CD227) was also positive, mainly in the granulosum layer of the epidermis in the wart. Individual IgD positive cells were seen, in areas close to the vessels under the wart. Factor XIIIa, CD79a and CD11c/CD18 were very positive, colocalizing under the wart in the inflammatory infiltrate [see Figure 1].

DISCUSSION

Verruca vulgaris are most often associated with HPV-2 infection, although these lesions may also be induced by HPV-4 and HPV-7 [1-4]. Keratinocytes react to human papillomavirus (HPV) infection by proliferating, resulting in different clinical manifestations including flat warts, common warts and filiform warts. The clinical presentation may vary according to the HPV type and anatomical site. Although warts are usually a self-limiting disease, some HPV subtypes may favor malignant changes including Bowenoid papulosis;

this disorder is characterized by multiple flat macules or patches in the genital area, which may or may not be pigmented [1-4].

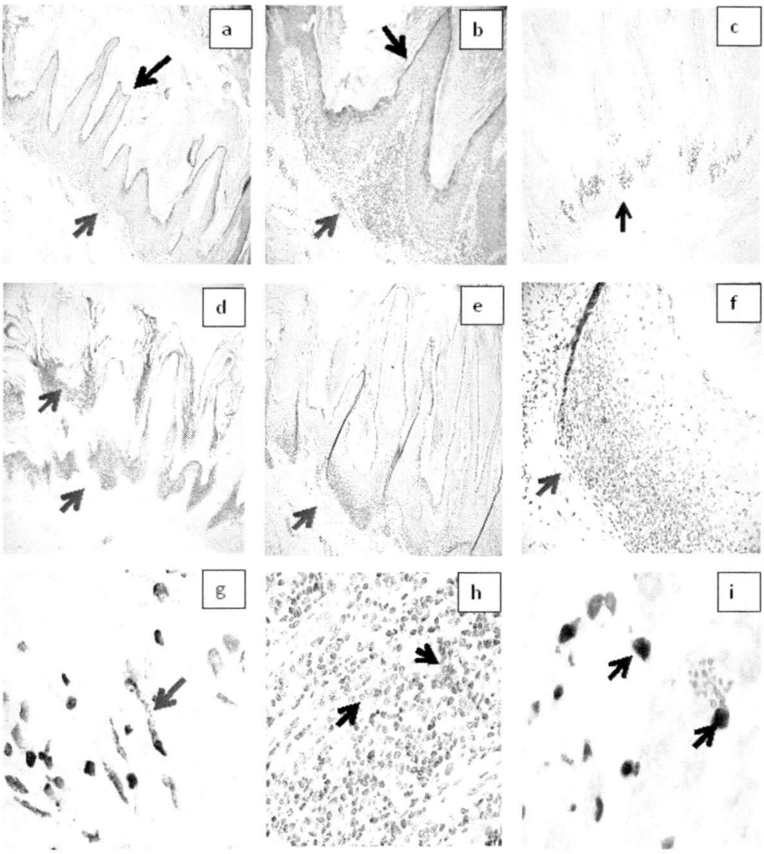

Figure 1. a and b H&E staining showing epidermal hyperkeratosis, papillomatosis, and hypergranulosis (black arrows) and an inflammatory infiltrate under the lesion in the upper dermis (red arrows) (40x and 100x, respectively). Note also inward projections of the epidermis, giving a curvilinear appearance to the lesional base. c. IHC positive staining with EMA/CD227 at the base of the wart (brown staining; black arrow) (40x). d. IHC positive staining within the upper and lower wart with Cytokeratin AE1/AE3 (brown staining; red arrows). e and f. IHC positive staining with CD11c, on inflammatory cells under the wart (pinkish staining; red arrows) (100x and 200x, respectively). g. IHC positive staining with IgD on some fibroblastoid cells in the upper dermis under the wart (pink-purple staining; red arrow) (400x). h. Double IHC staining on the inflammatory infiltrate under the wart with Factor XIIIa in brown, and CD79a in red (black arrows). i. IHC positive staining with Factor XIIIa, showing red-blue dark staining in the dermis under the wart (black arrows).

Other forms of superficial squamous cell carcinoma may be induced by HPV infection, including periungual Bowen's disease [1-4].

In our case, we found positive IHC staining on monocytes (CD11c/CD18/LFA), and B cell receptors (CD79a) as well as some antigen presenting dermal dendrocytes (Factor XIIIa). The CD11c/CD18/LFA-1 antigen is an integrin alpha X chain protein that is an integral membrane heterodimer protein, and composed of an alpha chain and a beta chain. CD11c is expressed by monoocytes, macrophages, neutrophils, myeloid dendritic cells and a small subset of lymphocytes [12]. The monoclonal antibodies to CD11c have proven especially useful in the diagnosis of several malignances such as hairy cell leukemia, systemic mastocytosis and lymphomas derived from histiocytes and/or dendritic cells; in our case, we found no signs of malignancy [12]. CD11c seems to play a role in in the adherence of neutrophils and monocytes to stimulated endothelial cells, and in the phagocytosis of complement coated molecules. Other functions of this molecule seem to play an important role in cytotoxic T cell killing, and in the induction of cellular activation. CD11c binds multiple ligands, including complement factor fragment C3b (a key component in innate immune defense), fibrinogen, CD54/ICAM and bacterial lipopolysaccharides [12]. CD11c/CD18 also induces cellular activation and helps trigger neutrophil respiratory burst [12]. Given our results, the body immune system was reacting strongly to the wart.

We also found positivity with the CD79a antigen, also known as B-cell antigen receptor complex-associated protein alpha chain and MB-1 membrane glycoprotein. CD79a is part of the B cell receptor signaling pathway [13]. The CD79a protein and the CD79b protein form a dimer associated with membrane-bound immunoglobulin on lymphocytes, thus forming the B cell antigen receptor (BCR) [13]. The dimer formation occurs in a similar manner to the association of CD3 with the T cell receptor, and enables the cell to respond to the presence of antigens on its surface [13]. BCR aggregation rapidly activates the Src family kinases, i.e., Lyn, Blk, Fyn, Syk and Btk tyrosine kinases; in addition, it activates other adaptor proteins such as CD19 and BLNK, and signaling enzymes such as PLCγ2, PI3K, Vav, GTPases, and transcription factors. These activations in turn result in changes in cell metabolism, gene expression, and cytoskeletal organization. The complexity of BCR signaling permits many distinct outcomes, including survival, tolerance (anergy), apoptosis, proliferation, and differentiation into antibody-producing cells or memory B cells. The outcome of the response is determined by the maturation state of the cell, the nature of the antigen, the magnitude and duration of BCR signaling, and signals from other receptors such as CD40, the

IL-21 receptor, and BAFF-R [13]. Some malignancies are also positive for CD79a, including selected lymphomas, leukemias, and breast cancers. Based on the activation of the BCR, and our observed positivity with IgD, we suggest that some specific immune response was mounted to the wart/virus components.

The human dermis contains dendritic cells which present a spectrum of IHC phenotypes, including staining with Factor XIIIa. Factor XIIIa is related to a blood coagulation factor involved in angiogenesis, the final stages of the clotting cascade and in wound healing [14]. In normal skin, Factor XIIIa is expressed in selected dermal dendrocytes (DDs) derived from the monocyte/macrophage cell lineage. DDs are located predominantly around the microvasculature in the adventitial dermis, at the dermal-epidermal junction, and around skin appendages. DDs are usually found as occasional single dermal cells, not within the epidermis [14]. Increased numbers of Factor XIIIa positive DDs are present in several cutaneous inflammatory and fibrotic conditions [14]. Factor XIIIa, as well as CD79a and CD11c, are also positive in some malignancies. In selected cases it helps to differentiate between dermatofibromas and other fibrohistiocytic entities, most notably dermatofibrosarcoma protuberans [14].

In conclusion, most warts are not malignant and some inflammatory response may be present as the organism attempts to eradicate the HPV. However, it is important to be alerting for cervical and anogenital squamous intraepithelial neoplasia, anogenital warts, or those associated with patients who may be under immunosuppression; in these cases, HPV infection may lead to precancerous lesions.

ACKNOWLEDGMENTS

Jonathan S. Jones, HT(ASCP) at Georgia Dermatopathology Associates provided excellent technical assistance.

Conflicts of Interest

None.

Funding

Georgia Dermatopathology Associates, Atlanta, Georgia, US.

References

[1] Jabłońska S, Majewski S, Obalek S, Orth G. Cutaneous warts. *Clin. Dermatol.* 1997;15:309-19.
[2] Tschandl P, Rosendahl C, Kittler H. Cutaneous human papillomavirus infection: manifestations and diagnosis. *Curr. Probl. Dermatol.* 2014;45:92-07.
[3] Cardoso JC, Calonje E. Cutaneous manifestations of human papillomaviruses: a review. *Acta Dermatovenerol. Alp. Pannonica Adriat.* 2011;20:145-44.
[4] Dunne EF, Park IU. HPV and HPV-associated diseases. *Infect Dis. Clin. North Am.* 2013;27:765-68.
[5] Abreu Velez AM. Yepes-Naranjo MM, Avila IC, Londoño ML, Googe PB, Velásquez-Velez JE, Velez ID, Upegui YA, Jimenez-Echavarria A, Mesa-Herrera NR, Yi H, Calle-Isaza J, Howard MS. Tissue inhibitor of metalloproteinase 1, Matrix metalloproteinase 9, αlpha-1 antitrypsin, metallothionein and urokinase type plasminogen activator receptor in skin biopsies from patients affected by autoimmune blistering diseases. *Our Dermatol. Online*. 2013; 4:275-80.
[6] Abreu Velez AM, Klein AD, Howard MS. Specific cutaneous histologic and Immunologic features in a case of early lupus erythematosus scarring alopecia. *Our Dermatol. Online*. 2013;4: 199-01.
[7] Abreu Velez AM, Avila IC, Howard MS. Immune response in a cutaneous allergic drug reaction secondary to imidapril, benazapril and metformin. *Our Dermatol. Online*, 2013; 4:192-95.
[8] Abreu Velez AM, Brown VM, Shipp L, Smoller BR, Howard MS. N-TRAPS, C-ANCAS in a vasculitis-lupus-scleroderma-panniculitis overlap syndrome. *Our Dermatol. Online*, 2013;4: 83-86.
[9] Abreu Velez AM, Jackson BL, Velasquez-Cantillo KL, Benavides-Alvarez AR, Howard MS. Merkel cell carcinoma versus metastatic small cell primary bronchogenic carcinoma. *Our Dermatol. Online*, 2013;4: 64-71.

[10] Abreu Velez AM, Howard MS. Neural reactivity detected by immunofluorescence in a patient with a localized blistering disease. *Our Dermatol. Online,* 2013;4 91-04.

[11] Abreu Velez AM, Klein AD, Howard MS. An allergic bullous drug reaction triggered by levofloxacin and trimethoprim/sulfamethoxazole mimicking an autoimmune blistering disease. *Our Dermatol. Online.* 2012;3:341-43.

[12] Mazzone A, Ricevuti G. Leukocyte CD11/CD18 integrins: biological and clinical relevance. *Haematologica.* 1995;80:161-65.

[13] Dal Porto JM, Gauld SB, Merrell KT, Mills D, Pugh-Bernard AE, Cambier J. B cell antigen receptor signaling. *Mol. Immunol.* 2004;41, 599–03.

[14] Quatresooz P, Paquet P, Hermanns-Lê T, Piérard GE. Molecular mapping of Factor XIIIa-enriched dendrocytes in the skin (Review). *Int. J. Mol. Med.* 2008;22:403-19.

In: Inflammatory Markers, Oncogenes … ISBN: 978-1-63484-303-4
Editor: Ana Maria Abreu Velez

Chapter 5

Squamous Cell Carcinoma Immunohistochemical Staining Reveals Lateral Satellitosis, Undetected via Hematoxylin and Eosin

Ana Maria Abreu Velez[1,*], MD, PhD, Yulieth Alexandra Upegui-Zapata[2], MSc and Michael S. Howard[1], MD

[1]Georgia Dermatopathology Associates, Atlanta, Georgia, US
[2]PECET, University of Antioquia, Medellin, Colombia, South America

Abstract

Context: Squamous cell carcinoma (SCC) is one of the most frequent cancers in humans. SCCs are thought to arise from multiple factors, including sun exposure; upregulation/downregulation of cell cycle tumor suppressor genes and/or oncogenes; exposure to carcinogenic substances; immune system changes related to aging, and selected genodermatoses

* Corresponding author: Ana Maria Abreu Velez, MD, PhD, Georgia Dermatopathology Associates, 1534 North Decatur Road., NE; Suite 206; Atlanta, Georgia 30307-1000 USA. E-mail: abreuvelez@yahoo.com, Telephone: (404) 371-0077, Toll Free: (877) 371-0027, Fax: (404) 371-1900.

such as xeroderma pigmentosum. Case report: A 82 year old female presented to the dermatologist for an erythematous, inflamed lesion on her nose.

Materials and methods: A skin biopsy of the lesion was obtained for hematoxylin and eosin (H&E) staining and for immunohistochemistry stains. *Results:* Examination of the H&E tissue sections demonstrated focal areas of full-thickness keratinocyte atypia within the epidermal stratum spinosum; the epidermal stratum corneum demonstrated focal parakeratosis, and solar elastosis was noted within the subjacent dermis. A lymphohystiocytic inflammatory infiltrate was noted in the dermis, subjacent to the epidermal lesion. IHC staining demonstrated positive staining within the dermal infiltrate for CD15, CD45, CD68, Factor XIIIa, cyclo-oxygenase 2 and minimal CD4. In addition, CD1a positive cells were noted around hair follicles near the lesion. The epidermal lesion stained positive for pancytokeratin AE1/AE3, and epithelial membrane antigen (EMA/CD227). The diagnosis of inflamed squamous cell carcinoma in situ (SCC) was established. Proliferative markers including proliferating cell nuclear antigen (PCNA), Cyclin D1 and Topoisomerase IIα were also positive in the areas where Cytokeratin AE1/AE3 and EMA/CD227 were positive. In addition, these cell cycle proliferation markers revealed likely lateral satellitosis of the tumor. *Conclusion:* In this case, we demonstrate that the inflammation of an existing SCC lesion may be associated with subtle satellite lesions. Our findings should be taken into consideration in selected treatment modalities, including MOHS surgery.

Keywords: squamous cell carcinoma, inflammation, CD15, CD45, pancytokeratin AE1/AE3, epithelial membrane antigen (EMA/CD227), MOHS surgery, PCNA

ABBREVIATIONS

SCC	Squamous cell carcinoma
H&E	hematoxylin and eosin
IHC	immunohistochemistry
COX-2	cyclo-oxygenase-2
EMA/CD227	epithelial membrane antigen
DAB	3,3-diaminobenzidine
Topo	Topoisomerase IIα
PNI	perineural invasion
PCNA	proliferating cell nuclear antigen

Introduction

Squamous cell carcinoma (SCC) and basal cell carcinoma (BCC) represent the two most common types of human non-melanoma skin cancer. Etiologically, SCC is a complex, multistage tumor that is characterized by molecular modifications; in normal skin, these modifications are regulated by multiple genetic and epigenetic mechanisms. Differentially expressed genes correlate with specific features of SCCs, including lesional cytokeratin types [1, 2]. Moreover, the relationship between skin cancer and the immune response is complex. Tumor immunosurveillance in the skin is not well understood in SCC [1, 2].

Case Report

An 82 year old female presented to the dermatologist with a lesion on her nose that had become inflamed over the last week. The patient had noted the lesion for several years, but consulted the physician regarding the recent inflammation. The lesional skin was biopsied and studied utilizing hematoxylin and eosin (H&E) staining, as well as immunohistochemistry (IHC) staining; all staining was performed as previously described [3-7].

Materials and Methods

Immunohistochemistry (IHC): We performed IHC utilizing multiple monoclonal and polyclonal antibodies from Dako (Carpinteria, California, USA). We utilized mouse anti-human; cyclo-oxygenase 2 (COX-2), clone CX-294; Pan cytokeratin AE1/AE3; anti-leukocyte common antigen (CD45), Clones 2B11 + PD7/26; Factor XIIIa; CD1a, clone 010; cyclin D1, clone EP12; proliferating cell nuclear antigen (PCNA), clone PC10; human epithelial antigen, clone Ber-EP4; Topoisomerase IIα (Topo), clone Ki-S1; CD4, clone 4B12; CD15; and CD68, clone EBM11. We also used a Factor XIIIa antibody from Leica/Novocastra.

Single color immunohistochemistry: For our IHC testing, we utilized a dual endogenous peroxidase blockage with the addition of a Dako Envision dual link (to assist in chromogen attachment). We then applied the chromogen 3,3-diaminobenzidine (DAB), and counterstained with hematoxylin. The samples were run in a Dako Autostainer Universal Staining System. Positive and negative controls were consistently performed. The staining was performed as previously described [3-7].

IHC double staining: These were performed utilizing a Leica (Buffalo Grove, Illinois, USA) double staining system. Specifically, for primary staining we utilized a Bond Max platform autostainer with bond polymer refined red detection DS9390, an alkaline phosphatase linker polymer and fast red chromogen (red staining). For our secondary staining, we utilized bond polymer refined detection DS9800, a horseradish peroxidase linker polymer and a DAB chromogen (brown staining). Positive and negative controls were consistently performed. The staining was performed as previously described [3-7].

RESULTS

H&E staining: Examination of the tissue sections demonstrated focal areas of full-thickness keratinocyte atypia within the epidermal stratum spinosum. No acantholysis was seen. The stratum corneum demonstrates focal parakeratosis, and solar elastosis was seen within the underlying dermal tissues. Focal tumoral ulceration was observed. A superficial, perivascular lymphohistiocytic dermal infiltrate was noted subjacent to the lesion [Figure 1].

IHC staining: Diffusely positive, membranous and cytoplasmic staining was noted on the tumor cells on review of the cytokeratin AE1/AE3 special stain. The staining was noted in the primary lesion, and also in the epidermis lateral to the lesion. Cytokeratin AE1/AE3 was also positive in dermal eccrine glands. Negative staining on these cells was noted on review of the Ber-EP4 special stain [Figures 1 and 2]. Cyclin D1 and Topoisomerase were positive in the tumor, and in areas of the epidermal granular cell layer lateral to the H&E primary tumor (satellite areas). These stains were negative in the ulcerated tumor areas. Of interest, Cyclin D1 was also positive in sebaceous glands under the tumor, as well as in some vascular endothelial cells under the tumor. The lesional epidermis and subjacent vessels also showed focally positive staining for CD15, COX-2, CD45 and CD68. Of interest, clusters of CD15 positive cells were positive in the tumor, and in the adjacent epidermis. CD68 colocalized in several areas with the CD15 and COX-2 positive cells. Factor XIIIa positive cells were seen under the tumor in the dermis.

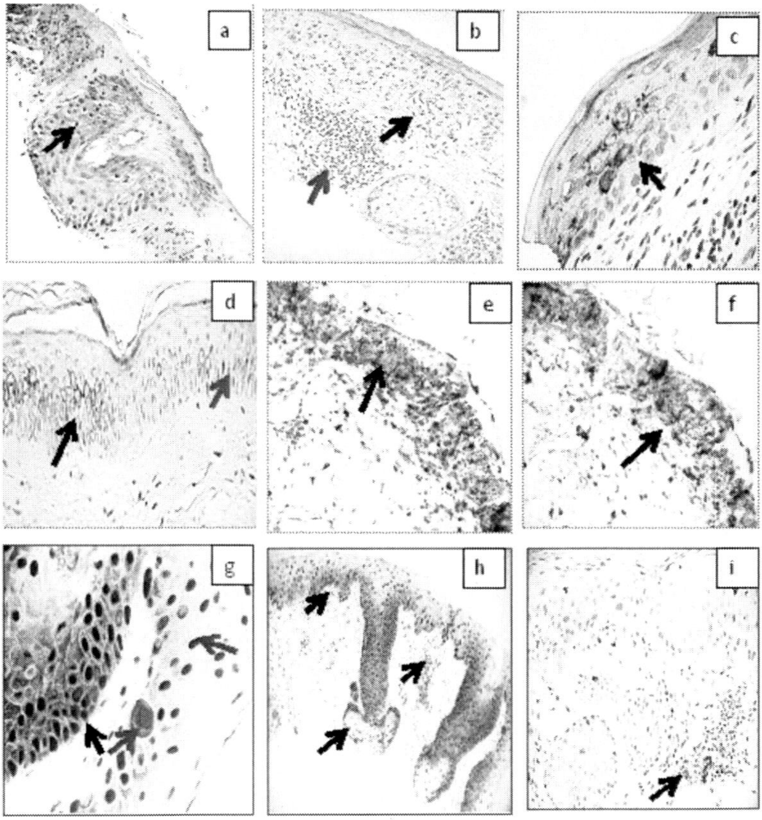

Figure 1. a and b. Show H&E staining at 100 and 200x magnification respectively, highlighting atypical epidermal keratinocytes(black arrows) and the inflammatory infiltrate under the SCCIS in the dermis (red arrow). c. IHC staining with Cytokeratin AE1/AE3 antibody, showing positive staining on atypical epidermal keratinocytes (brown staining; black arrow). d. IHC positive staining on the primary tumor atypical keratinocytes with Cytokeratin AE1/AE3 (brown staining; black arrow), and also lateral tumoral staining (brown staining; red arrow). e. Double IHC staining, using CD15(brown staining), and COX-2(red staining), showing overlapping staining in the inflammation in the affected epidermis(black arrow) and around some subjacent dermal vessels. f. Double IHC positive staining with CD15 (brown staining) and CD68 (red staining) in the epidermis (black arrow) and on subjacent dermal cells. g. IHC positive staining for PNCA, in the lesional epidermis (brown staining; black arrow). Please also note that in the adjacent epidermis, PCNA shows focally positive staining (brown staining; red arrows). h. Similar to g, but at lower magnification; demonstrating positivity of the PCNA marker in the epidermis, and also in subjacent dermal folliculo sebaceous units and eccrine ducts(brown staining; black arrows). i. CD1a positive staining in the lesional epidermis, sebaceous glands below the SCCs and around dermal blood vessels (brown staining; black arrow).

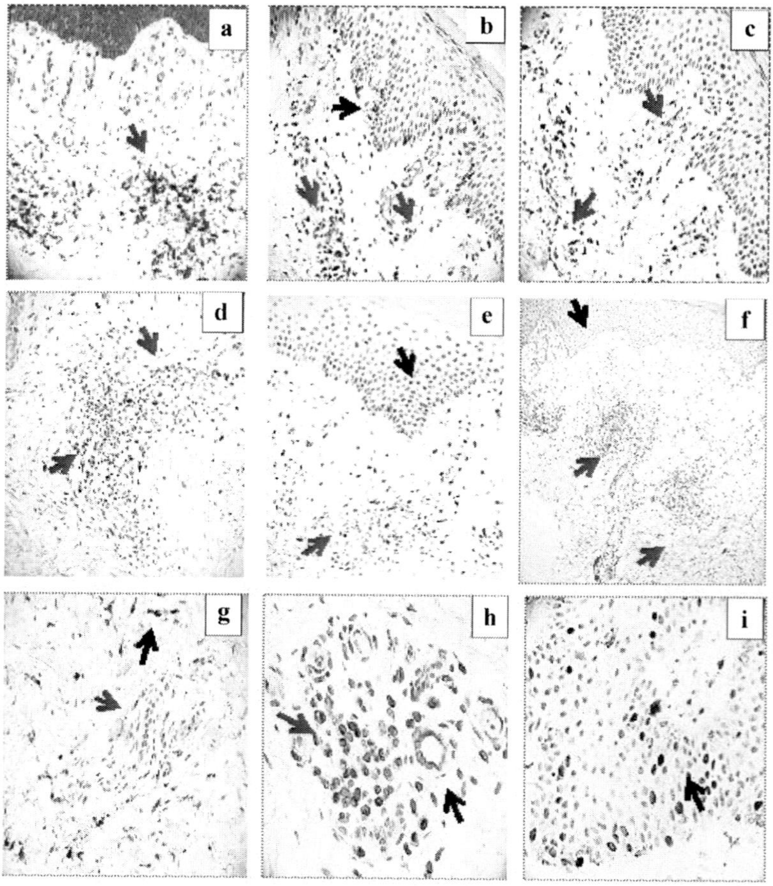

Figure 2. a. Positive IHC staining for cyclin D1 within the SCC (brown staining; blue arrow). Please note the additional, distant positive staining in a rete ridge area of the epidermis (brown staining; black arrow)(100X). The red arrow highlights positivity in a subjacent sebaceous gland(brown staining). b and c. Shows PCNA positive staining in the epidermis in the SCCIS, and also in the epidermis lateral to the H&E lesion (brown staining; black arrows). The red arrow shows positivity in a subjacent sebaceous gland (brown staining). In c, a higher magnification of the staining within the sebaceous gland (brown staining; black arrow). d. IHC positive staining for CD4, on cells in the dermis under the SCCIS (brown staining; black arrow). e. Positive IHC CD4 staining, around vessels close to the sebaceous gland (brown staining; black arrow, 400X). f, g and h. Positive IHC staining with CD15 in brown and COX-2 in red. In f, positive staining in the dermal infiltrate under the SCC (black arrows). In g, double staining within the SCC (black arrows). In h, double staining on the subjacent inflammatory infiltrate below SCCIS (black arrow) and only with COX-2 within the SCC (red arrow). i. IHC Positive IHC staining for Factor XIIIa in the inflammatory infiltrate subjacent to the SCCIS (brown staining; black arrow).

Contrary to Cyclin D1 and Topoisomerase, CD15, CD45 and CD68 markers were very positive in ulcerated area of the tumor. COX-2 was very positive in hair follicles in proximity to the tumor. Clusters of CD4 positive cells were seen around dermal vessels under the tumor [Figures 1 and 2]. PCNA was positive in the sebaceous glands under the tumor, as well as in some endothelial cells of the vessels under the tumor. PCNA was also positive in the tumor, and in areas of the epidermal granular cell layer lateral to the tumor (satellite areas). CD1a was very positive around vessels below the tumor, in the sebaceous gland under the tumor and in areas of the "apparently" normal epidermis around the tumor.

DISCUSSION

SCC is one of the most prevalent human cancers [1, 2]. It has been suggested that in SCC, tumor development is accompanied by an immune response that leads to tumor infiltration by inflammatory cells, and subsequent local and systemic production of cytokines, chemokines and other inflammatory mediators [8-11]. Studies in both human and animal models indicate that deficiencies in these inflammatory mediators may be associated with cancer progress [8-11]. Pancytokeratin AE1/AE3 and epithelial membrane antigen (EMA/CD227) represent excellent special stains for squamous cell carcinoma, in contradistinction to human epithelial antigen (Ber-EP4), which identifies the basaloid keratinocytes of basal cell carcinoma. Perineural invasion (PNI) is an important histologic finding in SCC, and represents a negative prognostic factor for SCC [12].

In our case, we demonstrate the strong presence of CD15 and CD45 positive cells infiltrating the SCC and its surrounding tissues. We also found inflammatory markers such COX-2, antigen presenting cells such as Langerhans cells (CD1a), CD68 positive non-Langerhans histiocytes and Factor XIIIa positive dermal dendrocytes. The ulcerated area of the tumor was strongly infiltrated by CD15, CD45 and CD68 positive cells, possibly indicating an immune system contribution to the ulceration. Such an action could in turn create a feed-back mechanism for recruiting more immune cells, possibly creating a self-augmenting/autocatalytic immune response.

Other authors have shown similar data to our findings. One group of authors studied T cell subsets (theophylline-sensitive T lymphocytes, and T gamma lymphocytes), and the activity of soluble immune response suppressor (SIRS) factor in 53 patients with SCC of the skin [13]. Eight of these cases had metastatic tumor in regional lymph nodes. The results showed decreased values for theophylline-sensitive T lymphocytes, and elevated values for T gamma cells. Tumor suppressor function evaluated by means of SIRS factor was normal in 36 patients with non-metastatic primary cutaneous SCC, and decreased in 8 with metastatic SCC [13].

We also demonstrated the presence of monocytes, macrophages and dermal dendrocytes among the cells infiltrating the inflamed SCC and in the surrounding tissues. Our results are similar to those of other authors, who studied the expression of Fc-IgG receptors on mononuclear phagocytes (monocytes/macrophages), as well as the activity of a soluble immune suppressor supernatant of T-cell proliferation (SISS-T) in 23 patients with SCC of the lower lip, including 8 patients with metastases in the regional lymph nodes [14]. The authors demonstrated a significant increase of the expression of Fc-IgG receptors only on circulating monocytes of patients with metastatic SCC. Tumor suppressor function evaluated by means of the SISS-T factor proved normal in patients with non-metastatic skin SCC, and decreased in 8 patients with metastatic SCC [14]. Dendritic cells (DCs) represent a diverse group of antigen-presenting cells, that link the innate and adaptive immune systems. DC capacity to initiate a robust and antigen-specific immune response has made them ideal candidates for cancer immunotherapies. Currently, the clinical impact of DC immunotherapy has been limited, which may partially be explained by the complex features of DC biology. Multiple distinct subsets of DCs have been identified in the skin, where they can be broadly subcategorized into 1) epidermal Langerhans cells, 2) myeloid-derived dermal dendritic cells (mDCs) and 3) plasmacytoid dendritic cells. Each subset is functionally unique, and may activate alternate branches of the immune system. These findings may be relevant for the treatment of squamous cell carcinoma, where others have shown that the tumor microenvironment may preferentially suppress the activity of mDCs, while LCs remain potent stimulators of immunity [14].

Other authors studied the expression of proliferating cell nuclear antigen (PCNA), a marker of cell proliferation, in 9 cases of pseudoepitheliomatous hyperplasia (PEH), 24 cases of keratoacanthoma (SCCKA), 47 cases of SCC and 5 cases of Bowen's disease (BD). It was observed that PCNA staining was marginal in PEH, SCCKA and well-differentiated SCC (WDSCC), and diffuse in poorly differentiated SCC (PDSCC) and BD [15]. The staining pattern of BD was unusual, in that the basal cells were often spared. While PCNA expression in PEH and SCCKA showed no significant difference from that of WDSCC, it was significantly different ($P < 0.05$) from that of PDSCC and BD.

The number of PCNA-positive cells in proliferating SCCKAs was more than that of regressing SCCKAs ($P < 0.05$). A positive correlation was noted between the extent of PCNA expression and increasing grade of invasive SCC [15]. The authors concluded that the distribution and extent of PCNA expression was closely similar among PEH, SCCKA and WDSCC, and also between PDSCC and BD; however, the biological behavior of entities within each group was different. They also concluded that PCNA was a good indicator of a proliferating cell pool [15]. As confirmed by our data, PCNA, cyclin D1 and Topoisomerase have been found by other authors to be excellent proliferation markers in SCC [16].

Our case details how an inflamed and ulcerated SCC interfaces with the host immune response to the tumor. Further studies are needed to confirm our findings. MOHS surgery is sometimes used in therapeutic removal of SCC [17]. Previous studies have addressed the SCC immune response and pertinent changes in expression of tumor supressor genes, oncogenes, cell proliferating agents and/or cell cycle regulatory molecules. These changes have been confirmed not only in the tumor, but also in peritumoral areas [18]. Due to our observed possible differences in biologic tumor borders defined via 1) H&E staining versus 2) proliferation marker immunohistochemistry, we suggest further studies of MOHS surgery versus larger resections for effective surgical therapy of SCC.

ACKNOWLEDGMENTS

Jonathan S. Jones, HT(ASCP) at Georgia Dermatopathology Associates provided excellent technical assistance.

Conflicts of Interest

None.

Funding

Georgia Dermatopathology Associates, Atlanta, Georgia, US.

REFERENCES

[1] Beer TW, Shepherd P, Theaker JM. Ber-EP4 and EMA aid in distinction of basal cell, squamous cell and basosquamous carcinomas of the skin. *Histopathology*, 2000;37:218-23.

[2] Guenther LC, Barber K, Searles GE, Lynde CW, Janiszewski P, Ashkenas J; Canadian Non-melanoma Skin Cancer Guidelines Committee. Non-melanoma Skin Cancer in Canada Chapter 1: Introduction to the Guidelines. *J. Cutan Med. Surg*. 2015;19:205-5.

[3] Abreu Velez AM, Howard WR, Howard MS. Upregulation of anti-human ribosomal protein S6-pS240, topoisomerase II ά, Cyclin D1, BCL-2 and anti-corneal antibodies in acute psoriasis. *Our Dermatol. Online*. 2011;3:113-17.

[4] Abreu Velez AM, Klein AD, Howard MS. Overexpression of linker for activated T cells, cyclooxygenase-2, CD1a, CD68 and myeloid/histiocyte antigen in an inflamed seborrheic keratosis. *North Am. J. Med. Sci*. 2011;3:161-63.

[5] Abreu Velez AM, Klein AD, Howard MS. LAT, EGFR-pY197, PCNL2, CDX2, HLA-DPDQDR, bromodeoxyuridine, JAM-A, and ezrin immunoreactants in a rubbed spongiotic dermatitis. *Our Dermatol. Online*. 2011;2:211-15.

[6] Abreu Velez AM, Klein AD, Howard MS. Junctional adhesion molecule overexpression in Kaposi varicelliform eruption skin lesions-as a possible herpes virus entry site. *North Am. J. Med. Sci*. 2010; 2:433-37.

[7] Abreu Velez AM, Smith JG Jr, Howard MS. Vimentin compartamentalization in discoid lupus. *North Am. J. Med. Sci*. 2010; 2:106-10.

[8] Sluyter R, Halliday GM: Infiltration by inflammatory cells required for solar-simulated ultraviolet radiation enhancement of skin tumor growth. *Cancer Immunol. Immunother* 2001,50:151-56.

[9] Pries R, Nitsch S, Wollenberg B: Role of cytokines in head and neck squamous cell carcinoma. *Expert Rev. Anticancer Ther*. 2006, 6:1195-03.

[10] Yanofsky VR, Mitsui H, Felsen D, Carucci JA. Understanding dendritic cells and their role in cutaneous carcinoma and cancer immunotherapy. *Clin. Dev. Immunol*. 2013;624123.

[11] Gasparoto TH, de Oliveira CE, de Freitas LT, Pinheiro CR, Ramos RN, da Silva et al. Inflammatory events during murine squamous cell carcinoma development. *J. Inflamm. (Lond)*. 2012;23; 9:6.

[12] Green JS, Tournas JA, Allen EJ, Youker SR, Fosko SW. Mohs frozen tissue sections in comparison to similar paraffin-embedded tissue sections in identifying perineural tumor invasion in cutaneous squamous cell carcinoma. *J. Am. Acad. Dermatol.* 2012;67: 113-21.

[13] Angelini G, Vena GA, D'Ovidio R, Lospalluti M, Meneghini CL. T cell subsets and soluble immune response suppressor (SIRS) factor in skin squamous cell carcinoma. *Acta Derm. Venereol.* 1983;63:109-14.

[14] Vena GA, Angelini G, D'Ovidio R, Pastore A, Meneghini CL.Monocyte Fc-IgG receptors expression and soluble suppressor factor in skin squamous cell carcinoma. *Acta Derm. Venereol.* 1983;63: 507-12.

[15] Li JI, Lee YS. Proliferating cell nuclear antigen (PCNA) expression in pseudoepitheliomatous hyperplasia, keratoacanthoma and squamous cell carcinoma of the skin. *Ann Acad. Med. Singapore.* 1996; 25: 526-30.

[16] Royds JA, Stephenson TJ, Silcocks PB, Bleehen SS. Proliferating cell nuclear antigen immunostaining in keratoacanthoma and squamous cell carcinoma of the skin. *Pathologica.* 1994;86:612-16.

[17] Gardner ES, Sumner WT, Cook JL. Predictable tissue shrinkage during frozen section histopathologic processing for Mohs micrographic surgery. *Dermatol. Sur.* 2001; 27: 813-18.

[18] Sansone P, Bromberg J: Environment, inflammation, and cancer. *Cur. Opin. Gen. Develop.* 2011, 21: 80-85.

In: Inflammatory Markers, Oncogenes … ISBN: 978-1-63484-303-4
Editor: Ana Maria Abreu Velez

Chapter 6

IMMUNOLOGIC AND CELL CYCLE REGULATORY MARKERS IN AN INFLAMED ACTINIC KERATOSIS

Ana Maria Abreu Velez[1,*], MD, PhD, Harry D. Vildibill[2], MD, FACS and Michael S. Howard[1], MD

[1]Georgia Dermatopathology Associates, Atlanta, Georgia, US
[2]Surgical Associates of Albany, Albany, Georgia, US

ABSTRACT

Inflammation of actinic keratoses (AK) has been described by some authors to appearing when these lesions become imminently precancerous, or in other instances when patients with specific internal cancers receive chemotherapeutic agents. Here we present a case of spontaneous inflammation of an AK, and investigate what type of immune reaction and cell cycle markers were present in the lesion. Case report: A 74 year old Caucasian female presented with a sudden erythema and itching in erythematous patches in her face. *Materials and Methods:* Skin biopsies were taken for hematoxylin and eosin (H&E) staining and

* Corresponding author: Ana Maria Abreu Velez, MD, PhD, Georgia Dermatopathology Associates, 1534 North Decatur Rd., NE; Suite 206; Atlanta, Georgia 30307-1000, USA, Telephone: (404) 371-0077, Toll Free: (877) 371-0027, Fax: (404) 371-1900, E-mail: abreuvelez@yahoo.com.

immunohistochemistry (IHC) staining; we studied many immunologic and cell cycle regulatory markers. *Results:* The H&E staining demonstrated focal atypia of the keratinocytes within the epidermis with hyperkeratosis, and focal parakeratosis. Within the dermis, an inflammatory infiltrate was observed of primarily lymphohistiocytic cells, clustered around dermal blood vessels subjacent to the AK. IHC staining demonstrated proliferation markers including Ki-67 antigen, topoisomerase II alpha, bromodeoxyuridine, proliferating cell nuclear antigen and thymidylate synthase; these markers were positive in the area of the inflamed keratosis, and also around subjacent dermal blood vessels. Inflammatory and antigen presenting cell markers such as CD3, CD4, CD8, CD45, S100, CD68, BCL-2, cyclooxygenase 2 and Factor XIIIa were positive along the basement membrane zone of the inflamed keratosis; some of these markers exhibited staining within the epidermis, and others were positive around dermal blood vessels subjacent to the AK. *Conclusion:* Our findings indicate that inflamed AK may have an important immune response, manifested via cell cycle proliferation markers within the epidermal lesion, the subjacent inflammatory infiltrate, and also in apparently normal skin around the AK. These results raise questions regarding MOHS surgery for persistent AKs, since some altered epidermal cells cannot be confirmed via routine H&E examination.

Keywords: inflamed actinic keratosis, MOHS surgery, cyclo-oxygenase 2, factor XIIIa, CD3, CD68, BCL-2, topoisomerase IIα, immunohistochemistry

Abbreviations and Acronyms

IHC	Immunohistochemistry
H&E	hematoxylin and eosin
BMZ	basement membrane zone
COX-2	cyclo-oxygenase 2
PDT	photodynamic therapy
AK	actinic keratoses
UV	ultraviolet
BCL-2	human B-cell lymphoma-2 oncoprotein
PCNA	proliferating cell nuclear antigen
Topo	topoisomerase IIα
Bromo	bromodeoxyuridine
TS	thymidylate synthase

ESA	epithelial specific antigen
SCC	squamous cell carcinoma
BCC	basal cell carcinoma
5-FU	5-fluorouracil

INTRODUCTION

Actinic keratoses (AKs), also named solar keratoses, are scaly, crusty patches that are considered precancerous; etiologic factors include ultraviolet (UV) light and genetic factors [1-8]. AKs are commonly seen in people with fair skin, blond or red hair, and blue, green and/or grey eyes [1-8]. AKs characteristically appear on sun-exposed areas such as the face, bald scalp, lips, backs of the hands; they are frequently elevated, "sandy" when palpated, and may resemble warts [1-8]. Often these lesions are erythematous, but some may appear pink, "brownish," and/or skin-toned. If left untreated, about ten percent of AKs may develop into squamous cell carcinoma (SCC), which is the second most common form of skin cancer [1-8]. Less frequently, AKs may precede development of basal cell carcinoma (BCC), the most common form of skin cancer. It has been estimated that more than 58 million people in the USA alone are affected with AKs. AKs are not only a medical problem, but also a very important esthetic issue for many patients [1-8]. Overall, accumulative and chronic exposure to UV light and living near the equator increases the likelihood of AK development. The incidence of AKs seem to be slightly higher in men, perhaps because men tend to spend more time in the sun and use less sun protection than women do [1-8]. Hispanics, Asians, African-Americans, and others with darker skin are not as vulnerable as Caucasians to AKs; however, AKs do present in these populations [1-8]. It has been suggested that when an AK become inflamed, it represents an early sign of transformation to squamous cell carcinoma (SCC), and/or less commonly to basal cell carcinoma (BCC) [1-8]. Sun damage in the skin is cumulative, so even a brief period in the sun adds to a lifetime total. Cloudy days do not provide complete protection, because 70-80 percent of solar ultraviolet (UV) rays can pass through clouds. The UV light emitted by the lamps in a tanning salon can be even more dangerous than the sun due to intensity, so dermatologists warn against indoor tanning. Occasionally, AKs may be caused by extensive exposure to X-rays or industrial chemicals. Because the total amount of time spent in the sun adds up year by year, older people are most likely to develop AK. However, nowadays, some individuals in their 20s are affected. Due to cumulative actinic damage, AKs are more common in people over the age of 50. Some experts believe that almost all Caucasians over 80 have AKs.

CASE REPORT

A 74 year old female presented with facial, erythematous, scaly plaques with itching_on sun-damaged skin. The lesional skin was biopsied and studied utilizing hematoxylin and eosin (H&E) staining, as well as via immunohistochemistry staining performed as previously described [9-14].

MATERIALS AND METHODS

Immunohistochemistry (IHC): We performed IHC utilizing multiple monoclonal and polyclonal antibodies from Dako (Carpinteria, California, USA), unless otherwise noted. We utilized 1) mouse anti-human B-cell lymphoma-2 oncoprotein (BCL-2), clone 124; 2) cyclooxygenase 2 (COX-2), clone CX-294; 3) von Willembrand factor; 4) bromodeoxyuridine (bromo), clone Bu20a, 5) CD20, clone L26; 6) CD45, leucocyte common antigen, clones 2B11 + PD7/26; 7) topoisomerase IIα (topo), clone Ki-S1; 8) CD4, clone 4B12; 9) CD8, clone C8/144B; 10) CD68, clone EBM11; 11) proliferating cell nuclear antigen (PCNA), clone PC10; 12) thymidylate synthase, clone(TS) TS106; 13) epithelial specific antigen (ESA)(Novocastra, 14) anti-human pancytokeratin, clone AE1/AE3; 15) Ki-67 antigen, clone MIB-1. We also utilized 16) polyclonal rabbit anti-S100. For our IHC testing, we utilized a dual endogenous peroxidase blockage, with the addition of a Dako Envision dual link (to assist in chromogen attachment). We then applied the chromogen 3,3-diaminobenzidine (DAB), and counterstained with hematoxylin. The samples were run in a Dako Autostainer Universal Staining System. Positive and negative controls were consistently performed. The staining was performed as previously described [9-14]. Finally, we utilized 17) Factor XIIIa antibody and 18) multikeratin from Novocastra.

IHC double staining: These were performed utilizing a Leica (Buffalo Grove, Illinois, USA) double staining system, as previously described [9-14]. Specifically, for primary staining we utilized a Bond Max platform autostainer with bond polymer refined Red detection DS9390, an alkaline phosphatase linker polymer and fast red chromogen (red staining). For our secondary staining, we utilized bond polymer refined detection DS9800, a horseradish peroxidase linker polymer and DAB chromogen (brown staining).

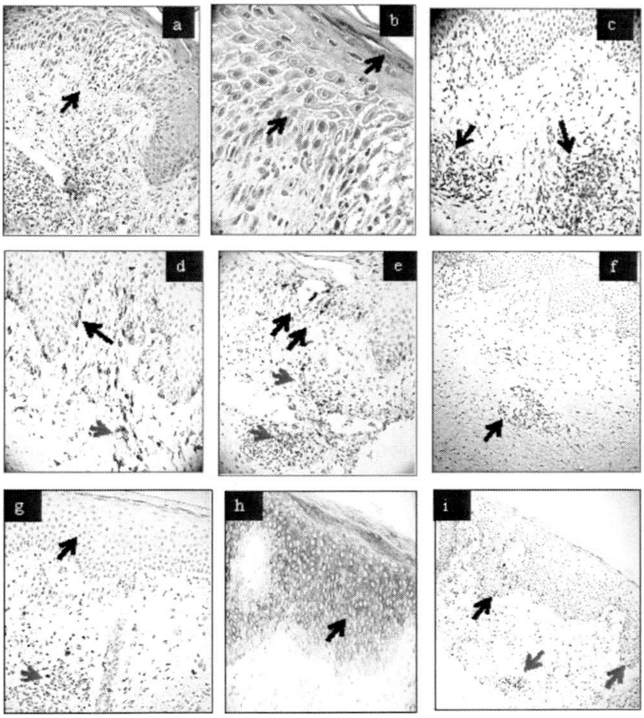

Figure 1. a and b. H & E staining at 100X and 200X, respectively. In a, focal epidermal edema is highlighted within the AK (black arrow). In b, actinically damaged epidermal keratinocytes and focal epidermal parakeratosis are highlighted (black arrows). c. Double IHC staining with CD4 in brown, and COX-2 in red showing double positivity in the inflammatory infiltrate around two dermal vessels under the AK (black arrows). d. IHC staining with CD45 positive cells along the BMZ in a linear fashion (brown staining; black arrow) and in the subjacent dermal infiltrate (brown staining; red arrow). e. IHC positive staining with S100 within the inflamed AK in the epidermis (brown staining; black arrows) and around subjacent vessels (brown staining; red arrows). f. IHC positive staining for CD68 in scattered dermal perivascular infiltrate cells (brown staining; black arrow). g. IHC positive staining for TS in the epidermis (brown staining; black arrow) and on inflammatory cells around dermal vessels (brown staining, red arrow). h. IHC positive staining with Cytokeratin AE1/AE3 in the AK (brown staining; black arrow). i. IHC positive staining with Topoisomerase in the AK (brown staining; black arrow), around dermal vessels and inflammatory infiltrate under the AK (brown staining; red arrow), and in an area lateral to the AK in the epidermis (brown staining; blue arrow).

RESULTS

Microscopic Description: A: Examination of the H&E tissue sections demonstrated focal atypia of the keratinocytes within the epidermis. Surface maturation was present. Overlying the epidermis, hyperkeratosis with focal parakeratosis was identified [Figure 1]. Within the dermis, a mild, superficial, perivascular infiltrate of lymphocytes and histiocytes was observed subjacent to the epidermal lesion. The lesion contacts the lateral specimen borders in the sections examined.

IHC STAINING

We found positive staining for several cell proliferation markers such as Ki-67 antigen, topoisomerase, proliferating cell nuclear antigen, topoisomerase, bromodeoxyuridine and TS overexpressed in the AK lesion, as well in the inflammatory cells under the AK and in satellite epidermal foci lateral to the primary lesion. Pancytokeratin AE1/AE3, ESA, CD3, CD4, CD8, CD45, CD68, S100, cyclo-oxygenase 2, BCL-2 and Factor XIIIa exhibited focally positive staining along the basement membrane zone of the primary inflamed keratosis, in selected cells infiltrating the epidermis and around blood vessels subjacent to the AK. BCL-2 staining was also very positive in the inflammatory infiltrate under the AK, associated with strong expression of von Willembrand factor in these vessels [Figures 1 and 2]. Topoisomerase, PCNA and bromodeoxyuridine were positive within the AK [Figures 1 and 2]. CD8 and Factor XIIIa were also positive around dermal eccrine gland ducts. CD20 was largely negative.

DISCUSSION

Ultraviolet light plays an important etiologic role in AKs; in addition, individuals whose immune defenses are weakened by cancer chemotherapy, AIDS or organ transplantation are more likely to develop AKs. Though only about 10 percent of AKs turn into cancers, there is no way to know in advance which ones will develop into carcinomas. Thus, many effective treatments are available for eliminating AKs [1-8, 15].

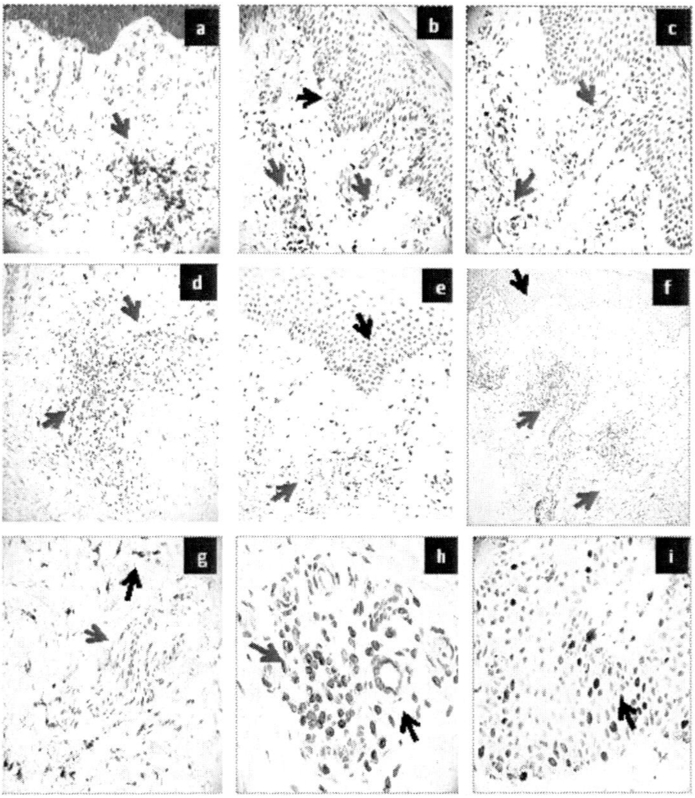

Figure 2. All IHC staining. a. Double IHC using anti-multikeratin (in red) and CD3 in brown, showing positive staining with multikeratin in the epidermis; CD3 staining is noted within the inflammatory infiltrate around dermal blood vessels (red arrow). b. BCl-2 (brown staining) and von Willembrand factor (red staining) colocalizing in the inflammatory infiltrate around dermal vessels under the AK (red arrows); BCL-2 is also positive along the BMZ (black arrow). c. Double IHC positive staining with Factor XIIIa (brown) and CD8 (red) overlapping in the dermal inflammatory infiltrate (red arrows). d. IHC positive staining with TS in red around dermal vessels (brown staining; red arrows). e. Positive IHC staining with PCNA in the epidermis (brown staining; black arrow) and in the infiltrate (brown staining; red arrow). f. Double IHC staining, with CD4 in brown and COX-2 in red overlapping around dermal vessels (red arrow; the black arrow shows positive stain in the epidermis with COX-2). g. Double IHC staining, using Factor XIIIa in red and CD8 in brown; shows positivity in the inflammatory infiltrate around the dermal eccrine gland duct (red arrow), and on some dermal cells (black arrow). h. Double IHC staining, using von Willembrand factor in red and BCL-2 in brown, and showing positivity in the inflammatory infiltrate(red arrow) around a dermal vessel (black arrow). i. IHC positive staining with Topoisomerase in the epidermis within the AK (brown staining; black arrow).

When an AK is suspected to be an early cancer, the physician may take tissue for a biopsy. The physician may shave off the top of the lesion with a scalpel, or scrape it off with a curette. The best way to prevent AKs is avoid direct sun exposure, especially in the middle of the day.

Photodynamic therapy (PDT) is a medical treatment that utilizes a photosensitizing molecule (frequently a drug that becomes activated by light exposure), and a light source to activate the applied drug. AKs and certain other types of cancer cells can be eliminated via this technique. There are a number of other effective treatments for eradicating actinic keratosis [15]. The treatments include cryosurgery, electrodessication and curettage, shave removal, chemical peels, topical imiquimoid and 5-fluorouracil. Solaraze gel is a non-steroidal medication, which also works fairly well on AKs. Treatment with Solaraze is twice daily for ninety days.

In our study, we found positivity with several cell cycle regulatory markers including bromodeoxyuridine, topoisomerase, proliferating cell nuclear antigen/PCNA, Ki-67, and thymidylate synthase. The positive markers were found not only within the AK, but also in inflammatory cells around dermal vessels under the AK, and in epidermal areas lateral to the AK. This indicates that the inflamed AK is exerting some type of cell proliferation effect on epidermal areas near the lesion, activating their cell proliferation. We found positivity in several cell cycle markers; the first marker was bromodeoxyuridine. The bromodeoxyuridine marker binds to cells that have incorporated bromodeoxyuridine into their DNA during the S phase of the cell cycle. We also found positivity with the topoisomerase II enzyme, that regulates DNA topology by cleaving and rejoining DNA strands, allowing other DNA strands to pass through the transient gaps. The topoisomerase IIα isoform is a 170 kDa nuclear protein, only expressed in proliferating cells. Furthermore, topoisomerase IIα is an important cellular target of several chemotherapeutic drugs. Third, we found positivity with thymidylate synthetase (TS); TS is a key enzyme in the synthesis of DNA. TS, along with the methyl donor 5,10-methylenetetrahydrofolate, catalyzes the methylation of deoxyuridine monophosphate (dUMP) to deoxythymidine monophosphate (dTMP) to generate the thymine nucleotides necessary for DNA biosynthesis. TS is also a target for fluorinated pyrimidine drugs such as therapeutic 5-fluorouracil (5-FU). The active metabolite of 5-FU, FdUMP, competes with dUMP for the active binding site on the TS enzyme. Our fourth positive proliferation marker, PCNA, is expressed by proliferating cells and reaches its maximum synthesis during the S-phase of the cell cycle. PCNA is a DNA clamp that acts as a processivity factor for DNA polymerase δ in eukaryotic cells and is essential for replication. The protein encoded by this gene is found in the nucleus and is a cofactor of DNA polymerase delta. The encoded protein acts as a homotrimer and helps increase the processivity of leading strand synthesis during DNA replication [16].

Factor XIIIa positive cells in human skin represent a specific population of bone marrow dermal dendritic cells, distinct from Langerhans cells; the dermal dendrocytes share some features common to mononuclear phagocytes. In benign skin conditions such as inflammatory dermatoses (eg, atopic eczema and psoriasis), an increased number of Factor XIIIa positive cells are present may in the upper dermis, closely associated with lymphocytes [17].

In conclusion, an inflamed actinic keratosis need to be treated to prevent conversion to squamous cell carcinoma; however, AKs elicit a defense immune response against the AK itself. Our findings also question the ability of MOHS surgery to accurately treat inflamed AKs, since regular H&E stains do not reveal the immunologically altered cells lateral to the H&E AK. In the inflamed AK immune response, many cells and structures around the H&E AK are altered as demonstrated by our positive IHC staining with multiple cellular proliferation markers.

Acknowledgments

Jonathan S. Jones, HT(ASCP) at Georgia Dermatopathology Associates provided excellent technical assistance.

Declarations of Conflicts of Interest

None.

Funding

Georgia Dermatopathology Associates.

REFERENCES

[1] Cantisani C, De Gado F, Ulrich M, Bottoni U, Iacobellis F, Richetta AG, Calvieri S. Actinic keratosis: review of the literature and new patents. *Recent Pat. Inflamm. Allergy Drug Discov.* 2013;7:168-75.

[2] Fenske NA, Spencer J, Adam F. Actinic keratoses: past, present and future. *J. Drugs Dermatol.* 2010;9:s45-49.

[3] Uhlenhake EE. Optimal treatment of actinic keratoses. *Clin. Interv. Aging.* 2013;8:29-35.

[4] Puizina-Ivić N, Mirić L, Carija A, Karlica D, Marasović D. Modern approach to topical treatment of aging skin. *Coll Antropol.* 2010;34:1145-43.

[5] Goldberg LH, Mamelak AJ. Review ofactinic keratosis. Part I: etiology, epidemiology and clinical presentation. *J. Drugs Dermatol.* 2010;9:1125-32.

[6] Feller L, Khammissa RA, Wood NH, Jadwat Y, Meyerov R, Lemmer J. Sunlight (actinic) keratosis: an update. *J. Prev. Med. Hyg.* 2009;50:217-20.

[7] Anwar J, Wrone DA, Kimyai-Asadi A, Alam M. The development of actinic keratosis into invasive squamous cell carcinoma: evidence and evolving classification schemes. *Clin. Dermatol.* 2004;22:189-96.

[8] Berhane T, Halliday GM, Cooke B, Barnetson RS. Inflammation is associated with progression of actinic keratoses to squamous cell carcinomas in humans. *Br. J. Dermatol.* 2002;146:810-15.

[9] Abreu Velez AM., Calle-Isaza J, Howard MS. Cyclo-oxygenase 2 is present in the majority of lesional skin from patients with autoimmune blistering diseases. *Our Dermatol. Online.* 2013; 4:476-78.

[10] Abreu Velez AM., Klein AD, Howard MS. Junctional adhesion molecule overexpression in Kaposi varicelliform eruption skin lesions-as a possible herpes virus entry site. *North Am. J. Med. Sci.* 2010;2:433-37.

[11] Abreu Velez AM., Jackson BL, Howard MS A. Deposition of immunoreactants in a cutaneous allergic drug reaction. *North Am. J. Med. Sci.* 2009;1:180-83.

[12] Abreu Velez AM., Smith JG Jr, Howard MS. Vimentin compartamentalization in discoid lupus. *North Am. J. Med. Sci.* 2010; 2:106-10.

[13] Abreu Velez AM., Howard MS, Brown VM. Halo nevus a complex immune response in halo nevi correlates with immune reactivity on

infiltrated melanocytes, adjacent hair follicles and blood vessels. *Our Derm. Online.* 2014;5:391-94.

[14] Abreu Velez AM., Howard MS, Pereyo NY, Delman KA, Mihm MC, Rizzo M. Lymphohistiocytic CD45/CD8 immune response in a case of malignant melanoma, with possible cannibalism. *North Am. J. Med. Sci;* 2012; 4:507-09.

[15] Dodds A, Chia A, Shumack S. Actinic keratosis: rationale and management. *Dermatol. Ther. (Heidelb).* 2014;4:11-21.

[16] Tsuji T, Kitajima S, Koashi Y. Expression of proliferating cell nuclear antigen (PCNA) and apoptosis related antigen in epithelial skin tumors. *Am. J. Dermatopathol.* 1998;20:164-69.

[17] Hermanns-Lê T, Uhoda I, Piérard-Franchimont C, Piérard GE. Factor XIII a-positive dermal dendrocytes and shear wave propagation in human skin. *Eur. J. Clin. Invest.* 2002;32:847-51.

In: Inflammatory Markers, Oncogenes ... ISBN: 978-1-63484-303-4
Editor: Ana Maria Abreu Velez

Chapter 7

Ribosomal Protein S6-PS240, CD45 and Cyclooxygenase-2 in an Inflamed Mildly Dysplastic Junctional Nevus

Ana Maria Abreu-Velez[1,*], MD, PhD, Charles J. Douchy[2], MD and Michael S. Howard[1], MD
[1]Georgia Dermatopathology Associates, Atlanta, Georgia, US
[2]North Atlanta Dermatology, Duluth, Georgia, US

Abstract

Context: Dysplastic nevi are atypical yet benign lesions, which may exhibit some clinical features of melanoma. They are characterized by cytologic atypia and architectural disorder among the lesional melanocytes. Here we present immunologic findings in a case of a dysplastic nevus (DN) with inflammatory changes. *Case report:* A 41 year old male presented to the dermatologist for evaluation of a pigmented lesion on his left arm. A skin biopsy was taken for hematoxylin and eosin (H&E) review, and for immunohistochemistry (IHC) staining. *Results:* H&E analysis confirmed histologic features of a dysplastic nevus. IHC staining was positive for ribosomal protein S6-

* Corresponding author: Ana Maria Abreu Velez, MD, PhD, Georgia Dermatopathology Associates, 1534 North Decatur Road., NE; Suite 206; Atlanta, Georgia 30307-1000 USA, Telephone: (404) 371-0077, Toll Free: (877) 371-0027, Fax: (404) 371-1900, E-mail: abreuvelez@yahoo.com.

ps240 and cyclooxygenase-2 not only in the lesion, but also in an inflammatory infiltrate around the subjacent dermal blood vessels. CD45 positive cells were also seen around vessels under the DN. *Conclusion:* Further study of cell signaling, inflammatory markers and immune response cells is warranted around dysplastic nevi, as demonstrated in this case in which the DN elicits a significant host immune response.

Case report: A 41 year old male presented to the dermatologist for evaluation of a pigmented lesion on his left arm. On clinical examination, the lesion was a large dark macule with a raised area at the center, presenting a scanning "fried egg" profile. The lesion displayed an array of several colors, ranging from pink to dark brown. The lesion was approximately 10 millimeters in diameter. A skin biopsy was obtained, and hematoxylin and eosin (H&E) and immunohistochemistry (IHC) staining was performed as previously described [5-7]. After the diagnosis was rendered, a surgical excision of the lesion was also performed.

Keywords: dysplastic nevi (DN), ribosomal protein S6-ps240, cyclooxygenase-2, CD45

ABBREVIATIONS

H&E	Hematoxylin and eosin
IHC	immunohistochemistry
DAB	3,3-diaminobenzidine
DN	dysplastic nevus
BMZ	basement membrane zone
Ribo	ribosomal protein S6-ps240
COX-2	cyclooxygenase-2

INTRODUCTION

A dysplastic nevus (DN) may be larger than a common mole, with atypical color, surface, and border features. The term atypical mole is sometimes utilized, instead of DN [1-4]. Atypical moles/dysplastic nevi are acquired melanocytic lesions of the skin with evolving clinical and histologic definitions. They are usually more than 5 millimeters in diameter, and may display a mixture of several colors; these colors range from pink to dark brown, and even black. Usually the lesion is flat with a smooth, slightly scaly or pebbly surface; it often has an irregular edge. A dysplastic nevus may occur anywhere on the body, but are usually noted in sun exposed areas [1-5].

Materials and Methods

Our hematoxylin and eosin (H&E) and immunohistochemistry (IHC) staining were performed as previously described [5-7].

Immunohistochemistry (IHC)

We performed IHC utilizing multiple monoclonal and polyclonal antibodies from Dako (Carpinteria, California, USA) as previously described [5-7]. We utilized 1) mouse anti-human ribosomal protein S6-pS240 phosphorylation site specific (Ribo), clone DAK-S6-240; 2) cyclooxygenase 2 (COX-2), clone CX-294, and 3) leukocyte common antigen (CD45) clones 2B11 + PD7/26. Positive and negative controls were consistently performed.

Results

Microscopic description: Examination of the H&E tissue sections demonstrated a melanocytic neoplasm, with melanocytes present as nests and single cells located along the dermal/epidermal junction at the basement membrane zone (BMZ) [Figure 1]. Mild cytologic atypia was seen within these cells, but pagetoid spread of melanocytes was not appreciated. Melanocytes displayed bridging between adjacent rete ridges; lamellar fibroplasia of dermal collagen was also present. The neoplastic process appeared free of the specimen margins in the sections examined.

IHC staining: IHC staining demonstrated positive staining with Ribonuclease S6-ps240 and COX-2 not only in the lesion, but also within the subjacent dermal perivascular inflammatory infiltrate. In addition, CD45 positive cells were also appreciated within the infiltrate [Figure 1].

Discussion

In dysplastic nevi, it has been suggested that ultraviolet radiation and other factors may be activating genes controlling cell-signaling pathways. In potentially malignant lesions, these signals may control many aspects of lesional progression.

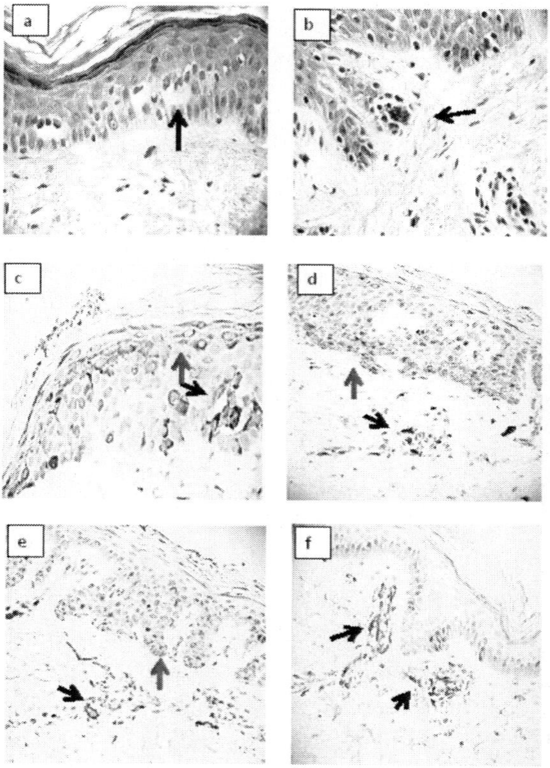

Figure 1. a and b. H & E staining, showing single and grouped melanocytes present along the dermal/epidermal junction (black arrow). The cells display mild cytologic atypia. In b, the lesion nested atypical melanocytes at an epidermal rete ridge tip (black arrow). c and d, IHC staining utilizing Ribonuclease S6-ps240. In c, positive staining in the epidermal stratum granulosum and spinosum layers over the DN (brown staining; red arrow) and also along the BMZ (brown staining; black arrow). In d, note positive staining along the BMZ (brown staining; red arrow) and in the inflammatory infiltrate around subjacent dermal vessels (brown staining; black arrow). e IHC positive staining with COX-2 not only in the lesion (brown staining; red arrow), but also in the subjacent infiltrate (brown staining; black arrow). f. IHC positive staining with CD45 in the subjacent infiltrate (brown staining; black arrows).

A recent trend has implicated COX-2, an inducible enzyme involved in the production of prostaglandins and thromboxanes in inflammation, in the progression of dysplastic nevi to malignancies. Previous authors retrospectively examined lesions throughout a spectrum of premalignant and malignant melanocytic lesions (dysplastic nevi $n = 10$, melanoma in situ $n = 4$, Clark Level II melanoma $n = 10$, Level III $n = 4$, Level IV $n = 3$, Level V $n = 2$, melanoma metastatic to lymph nodes $n = 13$, and melanoma metastatic to other sites $n = 3$) [8]. COX-2 was consistently observed in keratinocytes, dermal fibroblasts, and inflammatory cells in regions adjacent to dysplastic nevi and primary cutaneous melanomas [8]. However, contrary to our findings, the authors reported no COX-2 staining in the nevi themselves, nor in the primary melanoma tumor cells.

The authors reported that in addition, 13 out of 13 of the lymph node metastases expressed very high levels of COX-2 in overlying epithelium and inflammatory cells, and COX-2 was strongly detected in the metastatic melanoma cells *per se* [8]. The authors further detected COX-2 in several malignant melanoma cell lines. Like these authors, others have presented data suggesting that COX-2 may play a functional role in metastasis of melanoma, and concluded that melanomas express COX-2 significantly more than dysplastic nevi [9]. They suggested a test based on percentage fractions of COX-2-positive cells; the test would help in differentiation between early cutaneous melanoma versus nevi with high sensitivity and specificity [9]. However, there is only limited data regarding the exact role of COX-2 in melanoma pathogenesis.

In our own experience, we have observed noted the presence of COX- 2 as part of a nonspecific immune response. We have noted this specific immune response around and within lesions, in both keratinocytic and melanocytic premalignant to malignant progressions. We suggest that instead of forming part of the tumor progression *per se*, the expression of COX-2 may be part of a protective mechanism by the host immune system. Indeed, in the current study we clearly appreciated a CD45 response in areas near the dysplastic nevus. Moreover, how could a cell line of melanoma cells express COX-2? The answer may be that these cells were taken from fresh tissue that was expressing COX-2 as a host protective mechanism, in contradistinction to an invasive tumor mechanism expressing COX-2.

Ribosomal protein S6-ps240 kinase is a 90 kDa polypeptide 1 (RSK1; official name RPS6KA1) that has also been shown to be significantly hyperactivated in some human melanomas [10]. We do not know whether or not RSK1 was constitutively phosphorylated in these cases. S6-ps240 could thus act as a secondary cell signal activator and play a role in 1) stimulating gene expression and/or 2) promoting melanoma or other cell motilities, including among immune system cells.

We conclude that, given our findings, it is important to further investigate the dysplastic nevus microenvironment [11]. We suggest researching multiple dysplastic nevus cases for both specific immune response components, and any correlations with lesional progression.

Acknowledgments

Jonathan S. Jones, HT(ASCP) at Georgia Dermatopathology Associates provided excellent technical assistance.

Conflicts of Interest

None.

Funding

Georgia Dermatopathology Associates, Atlanta, Georgia, US.

References

[1] Clark WH Jr, Reimer RR, Greene M, Ainsworth AM, Mastrangelo MJ. Origin of familial malignant melanomas from heritable melanocytic lesions. "The B-K mole syndrome." *Arch. Dermatol.* 1978;114:732–38.

[2] Clark WH Jr. The dysplastic nevus syndrome. *Arch. Dermatol.* 1988;124:1207–10.

[3] Clark WH Jr, Elder DE, Guerry DIV, Epstein MN, Greene MH, Van Horn M. A study of tumor progression: the precursor lesions of superficial spreading and nodular melanoma. *Hum. Pathol.* 1984;15:1147–55.

[4] Clemente C, Cochran AJ, Elder DE, Levene A, MacKie RM, Mihm MC, et al. Histopathologic diagnosis of dysplastic nevi: concordance among

pathologists convened by the World Health Organization Melanoma Programme. *Hum. Pathol.* 1991.22:313-19.

[5] Abreu Velez AM, Howard MS, Hashimoto T. Palms with a polyclonal autoimmune response in patients affected by a new variant of endemic pemphigus foliaceus in Colombia, South America. *Eur. J. Dermatol.* 2010;20:74-81.

[6] Abreu Velez AM, Smith JG Jr, Howard MS. Neutrophil extracellular traps (NETS), IgD, myeloperoxidase (MPO) and antineutrophil cytoplasmic antibody (ANCA) associated vasculitides. *North Am. J. Med. Sci.* 2009;1:309-13.

[7] Howard MS, Yepes MM, Maldonado JG, Villa E, Jaramillo A, Botero J, Patino PJ, Hashimoto T. Abreu Velez AM. Broad histopathologic patterns of non-glabrous skin and glabrous skin from patients with a new variant of endemic pemphigus foliaceus (Part 1). *J. Cutan Pathol.* 2010;37:222-30.

[8] Goulet AC, Einsphar JG, Alberts DS, Beas A, Burk C, Bhattacharyya A, et al. Analysis of cyclooxygenase 2 (COX-2) expression during malignant melanoma progression. *Cancer Biol. Ther.* 2003;2:713-18.

[9] Kuźbicki Ł, Lange D, Strączyńska-Niemiec A, Chwirot BW. The value of cyclooxygenase-2 expression in differentiating between early melanomas and histopathologically difficult types of benign human skin lesions. *Melanoma Res.* 2012;22:70-76.

[10] Salhi A, Farhadian JA, Giles KM, Vega-Saenz de Miera E, Silva IP, Bourque C et al. RSK1 activation promotes invasion in nodular melanoma. *Am. J. Pathol.* 2015 ;185:704-06.

[11] Blaylock RL Cancer microenvironment, inflammation and cancer stem cells: A hypothesis for a paradigm change and new targets in cancer control. *Surg. Neurol. Int.* 2015; 29;6:92.

In: Inflammatory Markers, Oncogenes … ISBN: 978-1-63484-303-4
Editor: Ana Maria Abreu Velez

Chapter 8

Epidermis Above a Nodular Basal Cell Carcinoma Overexpressing Proliferating Cell Nuclear Antigen

Ana Maria Abreu Velez[1,*], MD, PhD, Billie L. Jackson[2], MD and Michael S. Howard[1], MD

[1]Georgia Dermatopathology Associates, Atlanta, Georgia, US
[2]Dermatologist, Macon, Georgia, US

Abstract

Context: Basal cell carcinoma (BBC) is one of the most frequently occurring cancers in humans. Contributory factors for the development of BCC include genetic predisposition, mutations, sun exposure, up/downregulation of tumor suppressor genes and oncogenes, overactive Hedgehog signaling, immune system changes related to aging and ionizing radiation secondary to radiotherapy. *Case report:* A 74 year old female presented to the dermatologist for an existing lesion on her right temple; on examination, the lesion consisted of a pearly nodule with telangiectasis. *Materials and methods:* A skin biopsy for hematoxylin and eosin (H&E) and for immunohistochemistry (IHC) staining was obtained.

---

* Corresponding author: Ana Maria Abreu Velez, MD, PhD., Georgia Dermatopathology Associates, 1534 North Decatur Road., NE; Suite 206; Atlanta, Georgia 30307-1000 USA.E-mail: abreuvelez@yahoo.com, Telephone: (404) 371-0077, Toll Free: (877) 371-0027, Fax: (404) 371-1900.

Results: Examination of the H&E tissue sections demonstrated a malignant neoplasm, comprised of focal aggregates of basaloid keratinocytes with hyperchromatic nuclei and minimal cytoplasm. Palisading of peripheral nuclei within the basaloid aggregates was also observed. Lymphohystiocitic inflammatory cells were seen in the dermis and vessels adjacent to the tumor. The histologic features were consistent with a diagnosis of nodular BCC. IHC demonstrated positive staining for proliferative nuclear antigen (PCNA) in the tumor, and also in the epidermis above the tumor; these epidermal areas did not show any abnormalities on H&E review. Of interest, other cell cycle regulatory and proliferative markers were also positive in the H&E normal epidermis above the tumor, including Topoisomerase IIα and Cyclin D1. Pancytokeratin (clone AE1/AE3) staining was positive in the epidermis above the tumor, but negative within the tumor. Human epithelial antigen (clone Ber-EP4) and EMA/CD227 were positive within the tumor, on lateral satellites of the tumor and in adjacent dermal structures. Conclusions: In our case, we demonstrate that an existing BCC may be associated with an immunologically directed immune response; that satellite BCC lesions need to be taken into consideration in treatment, and that multiple cell cycle and proliferation markers may be expressed distant to the primary BCC.

Keywords: basal cell carcinoma (BCC), inflammation, proliferating cell nuclear antigen (PCNA)

ABBREVIATIONS

BCC	Basal cell carcinoma
H&E	hematoxylin and eosin
IHC	immunohistochemistry
BCL-2	B cell lymphoma 2 gene
DAB	3,3-diaminobenzidine
PCNA	proliferating cell nuclear antigen
Ribo	ribosomal protein S6-ps240
Topo	Topoisomerase IIα
Ber-EP4	human epithelial antigen

Introduction

Basal cell carcinoma (BCC) represents the most common type of human cancer worldwide. Exposure to sunlight is one of the most important risk factors for development of BCC. Most, if not all, cases of BCC demonstrate overactive Hedgehog signaling [1-3]. The face is the most common area for BCC presentation. The primary clinical subtypes of BCC include nodular, superficial, infiltrating and morpheic. Combinations of these subtypes may occur in a single tumor. Sporadically, variable amounts of melanin pigment may be present within these tumors, which are then titled pigmented BCCs [1-3]. The primary histologic features of BCC include basaloid tumor cells budding from the epidermis or hair follicular units, peripheral palisading of nuclei in tumor nests, and focally mucinous stroma. Additional histologic subtypes include adenocystic (glandular differentiation), microcystic (milium formation), micronodular (often deeply infiltrating), neurotropic c(difficult to completely excise and frequently painful), and metatypical (includes some features of squamous cell carcinoma). The best immunohistochemistry stain for BCC is human epithelial antigen (clone Ber-EP4)[4]. Though it rarely results in death or metastatic disease, BCC can cause significant morbidity due to local tissue destruction. Management remains largely surgical, and includes electrodesiccation and curettage, surgical excision, and Mohs surgery. Topical therapies are effective for the treatment of some low risk BCCs [1-3]. A diversity of treatment modalities exist and are selected based on recurrence risk, tissue preservation, patient preference, and extent of disease. Cancer registries often do not collect data on BCC, so accurate prevalence and incidence is difficult to confirm. According to the American Cancer Society, more than 2 million people were treated in 2006 for non-melanoma skin cancer, mostly BCCs [1-3].

Case Report

A 74 year old female presented to the dermatologist with a slowly growing, pearly nodule on the right temple. The lesion contained linear telangiectasias, and an elevated, shiny border. A skin biopsy for histologic hematoxylin and eosin (H&E) and immunohistochemical (IHC) examination was obtained, and processed as previously described [5-12].

Materials and Methods

Immunohistochemistry (IHC): We performed IHC utilizing multiple monoclonal and polyclonal antibodies from Dako (Carpinteria, California, USA). We utilized mouse anti-human; Cyclin D1, clone EP12; Pancytokeratin, clone AE1/AE3; proliferating cell nuclear antigen (PCNA), clone PC10; human epithelial antigen, clone Ber-EP4; topoisomerase IIα (Topo), clone Ki-S1, phosphorylation site specific ribosomal protein S6-pS240 (Ribo), clone DAK-S6-240, and epithelial membrane antigen (EMA/CD227).

Single color immunohistochemistry: For our IHC testing, we utilized a dual endogenous peroxidase blockage, with the addition of a Dako Envision dual link (to assist in chromogen attachment). We then applied the chromogen 3,3-diaminobenzidine (DAB), and counterstained with hematoxylin. The samples were run in a Dako Autostainer Universal Staining System. Positive and negative controls were consistently performed. Our staining was performed as previously described [5-2].

IHC double staining: Our double staining was performed utilizing a Leica (Buffalo Grove, Illinois, USA) double staining system. Specifically, for primary staining we utilized a Bond Max platform autostainer with bond polymer refined Red detection DS9390, an alkaline phosphatase linker polymer and fast red chromogen (red staining). For our secondary staining, we utilized bond polymer refined detection DS9800, a horseradish peroxidase linker polymer and DAB chromogen (brown staining). Positive and negative controls were consistently performed. The staining was performed as previously described [5-12].

Results

Microscopic H&E results: Examination of the tissue sections demonstrated a malignant neoplasm, comprised of focal aggregates of basaloid keratinocytes with hyperchromatic nuclei and minimal cytoplasm. Palisading of peripheral nuclei within the basaloid aggregates was also observed [Figure 1].

IHC staining results: Diffusely positive, membranous and cytoplasmic staining was noted on the tumor cells on review of the Ber-EP4 special stain. The Cytokeratin AE1/AE3 special stain showed positivity in the epidermis above the BCC, but not within the BCC. PCNA, Cyclin D1 and Topo were positive in the epidermis suprajacent to the BCC, and on BCC satellite lesions [Figure 1]. IHC staining with Ribo was also significantly positive in the epidermis above the BCC.

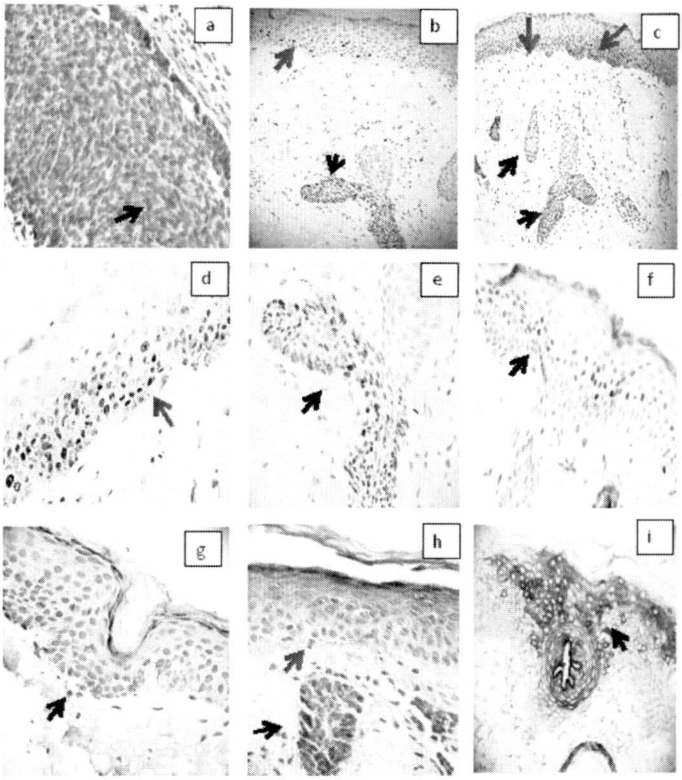

Figure 1. a. H&E staining shows focal aggregates of basaloid keratinocytes, with hyperchromatic nuclei and minimal cytoplasm. Palisading of peripheral nuclei within the basaloid aggregates was noted (black arrow) (10x). b through g, and i. IHC staining. b. Positive staining for Topoisomerase in one part of the BCC (brown staining; black arrow). Please notice that Topo is also positive in suprajacent basal layer cells of the epidermis (brown staining; red arrow). c, d, and e, Positive staining for PCNA in the tumor (black arrows) as well as in the epidermis above the tumor (red arrows). d Shows a highlight of the epidermal positivity at higher magnification (brown staining; red arrow). e. Shows PCNA positivity in the tumor (black arrow). f. Positive staining with Cyclin D1 on the epidermis over the tumor (black arrow). g. Positive staining with Ribo, mainly in the basal layer areas of the epidermis above the BCC (black arrow). h. H&E staining, showing a detail of the "apparently normal" epidermis (red arrow) and the BCC (black arrow) (400x). i. Shows positive staining for Cytokeratin AE1/AE3 in a proliferative area of the epidermis near the BCC (black arrow).

Discussion

BCCs can be classified into two broad categories on the basis of histopathologic features, namely indolent growth and aggressive growth subtypes. Indolent-growth subtypes include nodular and superficial [13].

We found that several markers that on increased expression show abnormalities in cell cycle regulation were positive in the BCC, as well as in the adjacent "normal" epidermis. Our results suggest that the tumor may be receiving and/or giving immunologic signals to the adjacent extracellular matrix and/or epidermis. We found strong expression of Ribo (a secondary cell signaling mediator) in the epidermis above the BCC; thus, we suggest that Ribo may play a role in BCC tumor proliferation. Further studies are needed to confirm this possibility.

The extracellular matrix (ECM) and the adjacent epidermis may play roles in invasiveness of BCC cells via adherence of tumor cells to ECM components. These tissues provide the matrix environment for BCC permeation, through the basal lamina and dermal connective tissue stroma.

Ber-EP4 is considered to be one of the best IHC markers for BCC, and indeed Ber-EP4 was positive on our tumor [14].

Other authors have shown that PCNA and other proliferative markers increase their expression in BCCs [15]. The authors used IHC stains for p53, PCNA and Ki-67 in superficial, nodular/noduloulcerative, sclerosing, infiltrative and metatypical BCCs, to determine whether the staining patterns differed in these histologic variants of BCC. Superficial BCCs were negative for p53 in four of eight tumors. Nodular BCCs showed moderately intense p53 nuclear staining with some peripheral accentuation. PCNA nuclear staining was greater than Ki-67, and fewer than 10% PCNA-positive cells were present in the nodular BCCs. Sclerosing and infiltrative BCCs showed intense p53 nuclear staining with peripheral accentuation. PCNA nuclear staining was greater than Ki-67, and PCNA positive cells were greater than 30% of the total cells in the majority of these tumors. Metatypical BCCs showed diffuse, intense p53 staining. PCNA nuclear staining was greater than Ki-67, and PCNA-positive cells were greater than 30% of the tumor cells in all metatypical tumors studied. The authors concluded that there were at least four distinctive patterns for staining for p53, PCNA, and Ki-67 that correlated with the different histologic variants of BCC [15].

As shown in our case, the epidermis adjacent to a BCC may show strong positivity for proliferative markers such as PCNA [16], Cyclin D1, and topoisomerase, even though H&E staining demonstrates normal histologic features in these areas. Our findings suggest that definition of surgical margins may need future redefinition in regard to treatment modalities such as Mohs surgery.

ACKNOWLEDGMENTS

Jonathan S. Jones, HT(ASCP) at Georgia Dermatopathology Associates provided excellent technical assistance.

Conflicts of Interest

None.

Funding

Georgia Dermatopathology Associates, Atlanta, Georgia, US.

REFERENCES

[1] Marzuka AG, Book SE. Basal Cell Carcinoma: Pathogenesis, Epidemiology, Clinical Features, Diagnosis, Histopathology, and Management. *Yale J. Biol. Med.* 2015;1:167-69.

[2] Cancer Facts & Figures 2010. *American Cancer Society* [Internet] Available from:http://www.cancer.org/research/cancerfactsstatistics/cancerfactsfigures2010/index .

[3] Rubin AI, Chen EH, Ratner D., Basal-Cell Carcinoma. *N. Engl. J. Med.* 2005; 353: 2262-69.

[4] Jimenez FJ, Burchette JL, Grichnik JM, Hitchcock MG. Ber-EP4 immunoreactivity in normal skin and cutaneous neoplasms. *Modern Pathology.* 1995;8: 8548.

[5] Abreu Velez AM, Yi H, Googe PB Jr, Mihm MC Jr, Howard MS. Autoantibodies to melanocytes and characterization of melanophages in patients affected by a new variant of endemic pemphigus foliaceus. *J. Cutan Pathol. 2011*;38: 710-29.

[6] Abreu Velez AM, Howard WR, Howard MS. Upregulation of anti-human ribosomal protein S6-pS240, topoisomerase II ά, Cyclin D1, BCL-2 and anti-corneal antibodies in acute psoriasis. *Our Dermatol. Online.* 2011;3: 113-17.

[7] Abreu Velez AM, Smith JG Jr, Howard MS. Subcorneal pustular dermatosis (Sneddon Wilkinson) with multiple immunoreactants. *Int. J. Clin. Exp. Pathol.* 2011;4: 526-29.

[8] Abreu Velez AM, Howard MS, Smoller BR. Antibodies to pilosebaceous units, in a new variant of pemphigus foliaceus. *Eur. J. Dermatol.* 2011;21: 371-75.

[9] Abreu Velez AM, Klein AD, Howard MS. Survivin, p53, MAC, complement/C3, fibrinogen and HLA-ABC within hair follicles in follicular degeneration syndrome. *North Am. J. Med. Sci.* 2011;3: 292-95.

[10] Abreu Velez AM, Brown VM, Howard MS. An inflamed trichilemmal (pilar) cyst: Not so simple? *North Am. J. Med. Sci.* 2011;3: 431-34.

[11] Abreu Velez AM, Jackson BL, Howard MS. Salt and pepper staining patterns for LAT, ZAP-70 and MUM-1 in a vasculitic bullous allergic drug eruption. *Our Dermatol. Online.* 2011;2: 211-15.

[12] Abreu Velez AM, Zhe J, Howard MS, Dudley SC. Heart immunoreactivity in patients affected by a new variant of endemic pemphigus foliaceus in El-Bagre, Colombia, South America. *J. Clin. Immunol.* 2011 ;31: 985-97.

[13] Sexton M, Jones DB, Maloney ME. Histologic pattern analysis of basal cell carcinoma. Study of a series of 1039 consecutive neoplasms. *J. Am. Acad. Dermatol.* 1990;23(6 Pt 1): 1118-26.

[14] Poniecka AW, Alexis JB. An immunohistochemical study of basal cell carcinoma and trichoepithelioma. *Am. J. Dermatopathol.* 1999;21 332-36.

[15] Barrett TL, Smith KJ, Hodge JJ, Butler R, Hall FW, Skelton HG. Immunohistochemical nuclear staining for p53, PCNA, and Ki-67 in different histologic variants of basal cell carcinoma. *J. Am. Acad. Dermatol.* 1997;37:430-37.

[16] Kurki P, Vanderlaan M, Dolbeare F, Gray J, Tan EM. Expression of proliferating cell nuclear antigen (PCNA)/cyclin during the cell cycle. *Exp. Cell Res.* 1986;166: 209-19.

In: Inflammatory Markers, Oncogenes ... ISBN: 978-1-63484-303-4
Editor: Ana Maria Abreu Velez

Chapter 9

EPIDERMAL TISSUE NEAR A BASAL CELL CARCINOMA OVEREXPRESSES PROLIFERATING CELL NUCLEAR ANTIGEN, CYCLIN D1, TOPOISOMERASE IIA, KI-67 AND P27^{KIP1}

Ana Maria Abreu Velez[1,*], MD, PhD, Billie L. Jackson[2], MD and Michael S. Howard[1], MD
[1]Georgia Dermatopathology Associates, Atlanta, Georgia, US
[2]Dermatologist, Macon, Georgia, US

ABSTRACT

Context: Basal cell carcinoma (BBC) is one of the most frequently occurring human cancers; scientific evidence demonstrates changed expression in cell cycle tumor suppressor genes and oncogenes. *Case report*: A 91 year old female presented to the dermatologist with a pearly nodule on her right arm with some telangiectasias. *Materials and methods:* A skin biopsy was performed for hematoxylin and eosin (H&E) and immunohistochemistry staining. *Results:* Examination of the H&E

* Corresponding author: Ana Maria Abreu Velez, MD, PhD, Georgia Dermatopathology Associates, 1534 North Decatur Road., NE; Suite 206; Atlanta, Georgia 30307-1000 USA. E-mail: abreuvelez@yahoo.com, Tel.: (404) 371-0077, Toll Free: (877) 371-0027, Fax: (404) 371-1900.

tissue sections demonstrated a malignant neoplasm comprised of focal aggregates of basaloid keratinocytes, with hyperchromatic nuclei and minimal cytoplasm. Palisading of peripheral nuclei within the basaloid aggregates is also observed. IHC staining demonstrated positive tumor staining with human epithelial antigen (Ber-EP4), establishing the diagnosis of a nodular subtype BCC. IHC staining with proliferating cell nuclear antigen (PCNA) was also positive in the tumor, and in the epidermis above and lateral to the tumor. IHC staining with topoisomerase IIα, cyclin D1, Ki-67 and $p27^{kip1}$ were positive in the tumor, and in the supposedly normal suprajacent and lateral epidermis. *Conclusion:* Multiple cell cycle regulatory markers were not only positive in the tumor, but also in the suprajacent and lateral epidermis; these areas were histologically normal on review of the H&E stain. These findings prompt us to ask whether surgical removal of BCCs may leave behind precancerous areas, only detected via IHC special staining.

Keywords: basal cell carcinoma (BBC), proliferating cell nuclear antigen (PCNA), cyclin D, topoisomerase Iiα

ABBREVIATIONS

BCC	Basal cell carcinoma
H&E	hematoxylin and eosin
IHC	immunohistochemistry
DAB	3,3-diaminobenzidine
PCNA	proliferating cell nuclear antigen
Topo	Topoisomerase IIα
Ber-EP4	human epithelial antigen

INTRODUCTION

Basal cell carcinoma is one of the most common human skin cancers; some variants are considered to be more aggressive, including infiltrative and morpheic subtypes [1]. Surgical excision is the "gold standard" treatment, with Mohs micrographic surgery (MMS) offering the highest cure rate. Other treatment modalities include photodynamic therapy (PDT) [2]. However, many recurrences after narrow surgical excisions and Mohs surgery have been attributed to perineural infiltration [3].

CASE REPORT

A 91 year old female presented to the dermatologist for a pearly nodule on her right arm with telangiectasias. A skin biopsy for hematoxylin and eosin (H&E) and for immunohistochemistry staining was taken. The H&E staining demonstrated a nodular subtype BCC, and the lesion was surgically removed.

MATERIALS AND METHODS

Immunohistochemistry (IHC): We performed IHC utilizing multiple monoclonal and polyclonal antibodies as previously described [4-7]. We utilized mouse anti-human cyclin D1, clone EP12; proliferating cell nuclear antigen (PCNA), clone PC10; human epithelial antigen, clone (Ber-EP4); CD68; topoisomerase IIα (Topo), clone Ki-S1; Ki-67 antigen, clone MIB-1; $p27^{kip1}$,'clone SX53G8 from Dako(Carpinteria, California, USA) and/or Leica/Novocastra(Buffalo Grove, Illinois, USA). PNL2 was use from Cell Marque Sigma Aldrich.

Single color immunohistochemistry: For our IHC testing, we utilized a dual endogenous peroxidase blockage, with the addition of a Dako Envision dual link (to assist in chromogen attachment). We then applied the chromogen 3,3-diaminobenzidine (DAB), and counterstained with hematoxylin. The samples were run in a Dako Autostainer Universal Staining System. Positive and negative controls were consistently performed. The staining was performed as previously described [4-7].

RESULTS

Microscopic description of H&E staining: Examination of the tissue sections demonstrated a malignant neoplasm comprised of focal aggregates of basaloid keratinocytes, with hyperchromatic nuclei and minimal cytoplasm. Palisading of peripheral nuclei within the basaloid aggregates was also observed [Figure 1]. The lesion contacted the true deep specimen borders in the sections examined.

IHC staining: Diffusely positive, membranous and cytoplasmic staining was noted on the tumor cells on review of the Ber-EP4 special stain in the tumor, but not in the adjacent epidermis.

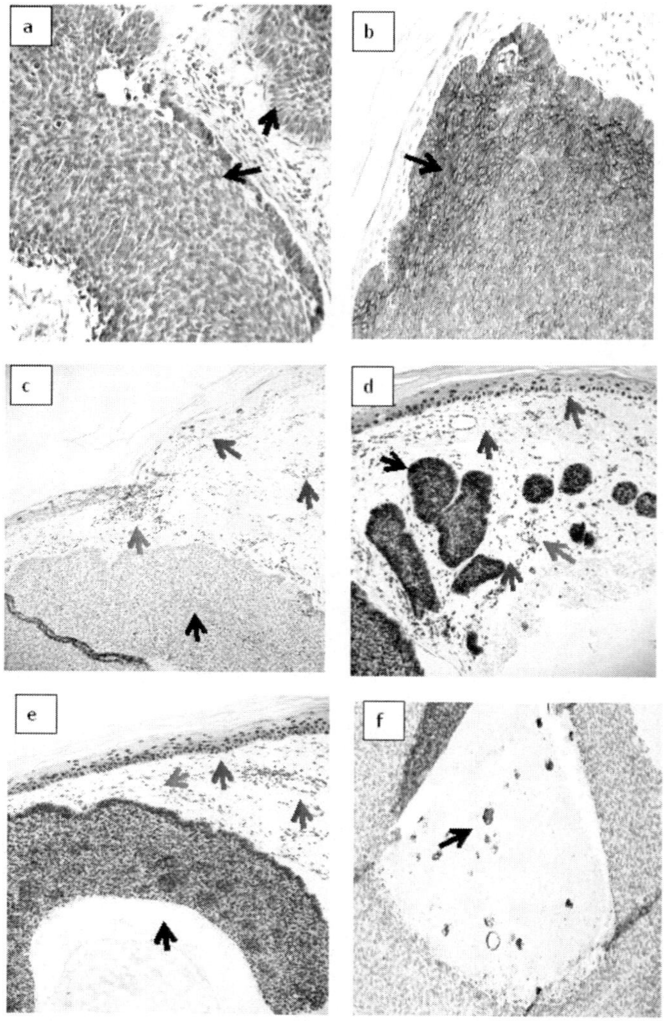

Figure 1. a. H&E staining, showing the classic morphology of a nodular BCC (black arrows) (200X). b. IHC positive staining with Ber-EP4 on the BCC (brown staining; black arrow). c. IHC positive staining with P27 in some parts of the tumor (brown staining; black arrow) as well as on adjacent inflammatory cells (green arrow), adjacent blood vessels (brown staining; purple arrow), and in the adjacent epidermis (brown staining; red arrow). c, d and e. Positive staining with PCNA at lower and higher magnification respectively, showing positive staining in the adjacent epidermis (brown staining; red arrows), in the tumor (brown staining; black arrows), on nearby blood vessels(brown staining; purple arrows), and on inflammatory cells around the tumor(brown staining; green arrows). f. IHC positive staining CD68 in a comedo necrosis area of a BCC lobule (brown staining; black arrow).

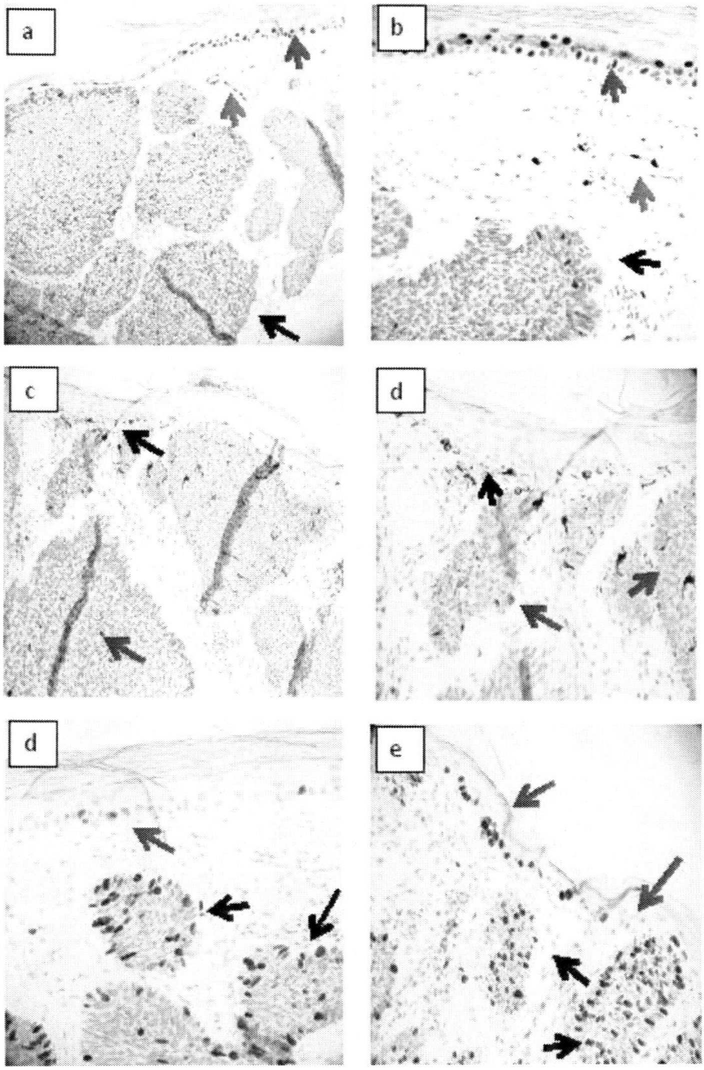

Figure 2. a and b. IHC staining with cyclin D1 in the tumor (brown staining; black arrows) as well as in the adjacent epidermis (brown staining; red arrows) and on adjacent blood vessels(brown staining; green arrows) at low and high power, respectively. c and d, IHC staining for PNL2, a melanocytic marker. Note the positive staining at lower (40X) and higher magnification (100X) respectively on melanocytes in the basement membrane zone of the skin (brown staining; black arrows), and inside BCC tumor lobules (brown staining; red arrows). e and f. IHC positive staining for Ki-67, showing positivity in the tumor (brown staining; black arrows), and also in some cells in the adjacent epidermis (brown staining; red arrows).

Proliferative nuclear antigen (PCNA) was also positive in the tumor, but also in the epidermis above and lateral to the tumor. IHC staining with topoisomerase IIα, cyclin D and Ki-67 was positive in the tumor, and in the suprajacent and lateral epidermis [Figures 1 and 2]. IHC staining with p27 was positive in the inflammatory cells around the tumor. CD68 staining was positive in a few histiocytic inflammatory cells around the BCC, and in comedo necrosis areas within the BCC.

DISCUSSION

One of the best known IHC markers for BCC is Ber-EP4, representing an antibody raised against a basaloid keratinocyte membrane glycoprotein of unknown function [8, 9].

Other authors have utilized proliferative and apoptotic markers including p53, bcl-2 and Ki-67 to correlate histologic findings and tumor aggression in BCCs [1]. These authors studied samples of the nodular, superficial and morpheic types of BCC and found that Bcl-2 expression correlated significantly with BCC aggression (in morpheic and nodular types). The authors also found that Ki-67, due to its variable staining patterns, could not be considered a reliable marker of aggression in BCCs. They also suggested that, based on their data, PCNA was not a reliable marker of cell proliferation in BCCs [1].

In our case, we found positive PCNA positive staining in the tumor; however the epidermis above and lateral to the tumor also stained positive. Similar findings were found with Topo and cyclin D1, that represent proliferative and cell cycle regulatory markers, respectively [9]. Our findings indicate that the tumor is interacting with the surrounding epidermis, and that adjacent stromal structures may contribute to tumor growth, invasive behavior and development of ectopic microtumors [10].

$p27^{kip1}$ also known as CDKN1B, CDK inhibitor and $p27^{kip1}$ is a critical regulator of cell cycle progression [9]; its positivity in the tumor, the surrounding epidermis and within adjacent inflammatory cells and blood vessels reinforces the concept that tumor growth is not an event exclusively involving the BCC tumor.

We observed some form of immune response in the comedo necrotic centers of some of the BCC lobules, where CD68 positive cells were seen. Our findings may indicate some kind of immune response causing tumor involution; however, larger studies are needed to confirm this possibility.

We conclude that the recurrence of BCCs in areas of proximity to a previously excised tumor may be explained by the ectopic expression of multiple cell proliferation and/or cell cycle regulatory markers; these findings are not present on classical frozen section and permanent H&E review. Further studies are warranted to confirm our findings, and to explore the role of these markers in permanent BCC removal.

ACKNOWLEDGMENTS

Jonathan S. Jones, HT(ASCP) at Georgia Dermatopathology Associates provided excellent technical assistance.

Conflicts of Interest

None.

Funding

Georgia Dermatopathology Associates, Atlanta, Georgia, US.

REFERENCES

[1] Corrêa Mde P, Ferreira AP, Gollner AM, Rodrigues MF, Guerra MC. Marker expression of cell proliferation and apoptosis in basal cell carcinoma. *An. Bras. Dermatol*. 2009;84: 606-14.

[2] Al-Niaimi F, Sheth N, Kurwa HA, Mallipeddi R. Photodynamic Therapy Followed by Mohs Micrographic Surgery, Compared to Mohs Micrographic Surgery Alone for the Treatment of Basal Cell Carcinoma: Results of a Pilot Single-Blinded Randomized Controlled Trial. *J. Cutan Aesthet Surg*. 2015;8: 88-91.

[3] Català A, Garces JR, Alegre M, Gich IJ, Puig L. Mohs micrographic surgery for basal cell carcinomas: results of a Spanish retrospective study and Kaplan–Meier survival analysis of tumour recurrence. *J. Eur. Acad. Dermatol. Venereol*. 2014;28:1363-69.

[4] Abreu Velez, AM, Velazques-Velez, JE, Howard, MS. (2015). Bullous Pemphigoid: Broader Concepts. In *Advances in Dermatology Research* (pp. 9-32). S.l., New York: Nova Science.

[5] Abreu Velez AM., Velazques-Velez JE, Howard MS. (2015). Dermal neurovascular structures demonstrate autoimmune reactivity in lesional skin of a patient with bullous pemphigoid. In:, *Advances in Dermatology Research* (pp. 33-44). S.I., New York: Nova Science.

[6] Abreu Velez AM, Brown VM, Howard MS. A bullous pemphigoid-like allergic drug reaction, with clues for differentiation versus classic bullous pemphigoid. In: *Advances in Dermatology Research* (pp. 57-66). S.I., New York: Nova Science.

[7] Abreu Velez AM., Jackson BL, Howard MS. Expression of Immunologic markers varies between intact blister and traumatized blister areas in a patient with bullous pemphigoid. In: *Advances in Dermatology Research* (pp. 45-56). S.I., New York: Nova Science.

[8] Jimenez FJ, Burchette JL, Grichnik JM, Hitchcock MG. Ber-EP4 immunoreactivity in normal skin and cutaneous neoplasms. *Modern Pathology. 1995;8: 854-58.*

[9] *Abreu Velez* AM, Howard MS. Tumor-suppressor Genes, Cell Cycle Regulatory Checkpoints, and the Skin. *N. Am. J. Med. Sci.* 2015;7:176-78.

[10] Mirancea N, Moroşanu AM, Mirancea GV, Juravle FD, Mănoiu VS. Infrastructure of the telocytes from tumor stroma in skin basal and squamous cell carcinomas. *Rom. J. Morphol. Embryol.* 2013;54:1025-27.

In: Inflammatory Markers, Oncogenes … ISBN: 978-1-63484-303-4
Editor: Ana Maria Abreu Velez

Chapter 10

Directed Host Immune Response against a Primary Cutaneous Squamous Cell Carcinoma

Ana Maria Abreu Velez[1,*], MD, PhD, Vickie M. Brown[2] and Michael S. Howard[1], MD

[1]Georgia Dermatopathology Associates, Atlanta, Georgia, US
[2]FamilyDermatology, Milledgeville, Georgia, US

Abstract

Context: Cutaneous squamous cell carcinoma (SCC) is the second most common form of skin cancer. These lesions feature uncontrolled growth of abnormal epidermal spinous layer keratinocytes, which comprise most of the epidermis. *Case report:* A 65 year old female presented to the dermatologist for a persistent, scaly red patch on her right arm with irregular borders; the lesion occasionally crusted or bled. *Materials and methods:* A lesional skin biopsy was taken for hematoxylin and eosin (H&E) review, and for immunohistochemistry (IHC) staining. *Results:* The H&E staining demonstrated a malignant keratinocytic neoplasm originating from the epidermis, and invading the subjacent

* Corresponding author: Ana Maria Abreu Velez, MD, PhD, Georgia Dermatopathology Associates, 1534 North Decatur Road., NE; Suite 206; Atlanta, Georgia 30307-1000 USA. E-mail: abreuvelez@yahoo.com, Tel: (404) 371-0077, Toll Free: (877) 371-0027, Fax: (404) 371-1900.

dermal tissues. Individual tumor cells displayed atypical nuclear features, with occasional mitotic figures and extensive keratinization. A diagnosis of primary cutaneous SCC was established. IHC staining showed an active immune response, with the presence of many antigen presenting cells; these included histiocytic cells displaying positive staining for CD68, HAM-56 and Factor XIIIa. In addition, T lymphocytes were present within the infiltrate, demonstrating positive staining for CD4, CD8 and CD45. BCL-2 positive cells were also positive in the inflammatory infiltrate. Conclusion: We found an active, robust and directed immune response in this SCC. Further, larger studies are needed to take therapeutic advantage of such an immune response.

Keywords: cutaneous squamous cell carcinoma (SCC), inflammation, immune response, HLA-DPDQDR

ABBREVIATIONS

SCC	Cutanous squamous cell carcinoma
H&E	hematoxylin and eosin
IHC	immunohistochemistry
BCL-2	B-cell lymphoma 2 gene
MHCs	major histocompatibility complexes
TCRs	T-cell receptors
PEP	peplomycin

INTRODUCTION

Primary cutaneous squamous cell carcinoma (SCC) is the second most common form of skin cancer. These lesions feature uncontrolled growth of abnormal cells arising in the epidermal spinous layer keratinocytes, which comprise most of the epidermis. Squamous cell carcinomas are at least twice as frequent in men than in women, partly because of more sun exposure in male patients [1]. Most SCCs appear in patients over age 50, but in recent years more patients aged 20 to 40 are being diagnosed with the disease [1]. Primary cutaneous SCC often presents as scaly, erythematous patches, open sores, elevated growths with a central depression, or wart-like growths; they may crust or bleed. SCC may become disfiguring and fatal if left untreated. An estimated 700,000 cases of primary cutaneous SCC are diagnosed each year in the US, and between 3,980 and 8,830 people died from the disease in the US in 2012. Recent data suggest the importance of studying regional sentinel lymph nodes in high risk SCC patients [1].

MATERIALS AND METHODS

A skin biopsy for hematoxylin and eosin (H&E) review and immunohistochemistry (IHC) staining was processed as previously described [2-5].

Immunohistochemistry (IHC): We performed IHC utilizing multiple monoclonal and polyclonal antibodies from Dako (Carpinteria, California, USA) as previously described [2-5]. We utilized CD68, clone EBM11; CD4, clone 4B12; CD8, clone C8/144B; CD15; CD57 and cytokeratin, clone AE1/AE3. HAM-56 was obtained from Cell Marque (Rocklin, California, USA). The following antibodies were utilized from Leica/Novocastra (Buffalo Grove, Illinois, USA): Factor XIIIa; epithelial membrane antigen (EMA/CD227), clone E29, and HLA-DPDQDR antigen, clone CR3/43. Positive and negative controls were consistently performed.

IHC double staining: These were performed utilizing a Leica (Buffalo Grove, Illinois, USA) double staining system, as previously described [9-14]. Specifically, for primary staining we utilized a Bond Max platform autostainer with bond polymer refined red detection DS9390, an alkaline phosphatase linker polymer and fast red chromogen (red staining). For our secondary staining, we utilized bond polymer refined brown detection DS9800, a horseradish peroxidase linker polymer and DAB chromogen (brown staining).

RESULTS

Microscopic Description: Examination of the tissue sections demonstrated a malignant keratinocytic neoplasm originating from the epidermis, and invading the subjacent dermal tissues. No adipose tissue involvement was noted. Individual tumor cells displayed atypical nuclear features, with occasional mitotic figures also present [Figure 1]. Extensive keratinization was seen within the neoplasm. No tumoral ulceration was noted. No acantholysis was seen [Figure 1]. No tumor cell perineural or perivascular invasion was appreciated. The tumor Broders grade was estimated at II/IV. The lesional depth of invasion was measured at 1.50 mm. The lesion contacted the deep specimen borders in the sections examined.

IHC staining: CD15 and Ber-EP4 were both negative on the tumor cells. Pancytokeratin AE1/AE3 staining was positive in the tumor, as well as on the normal epidermis surrounding the SCC.

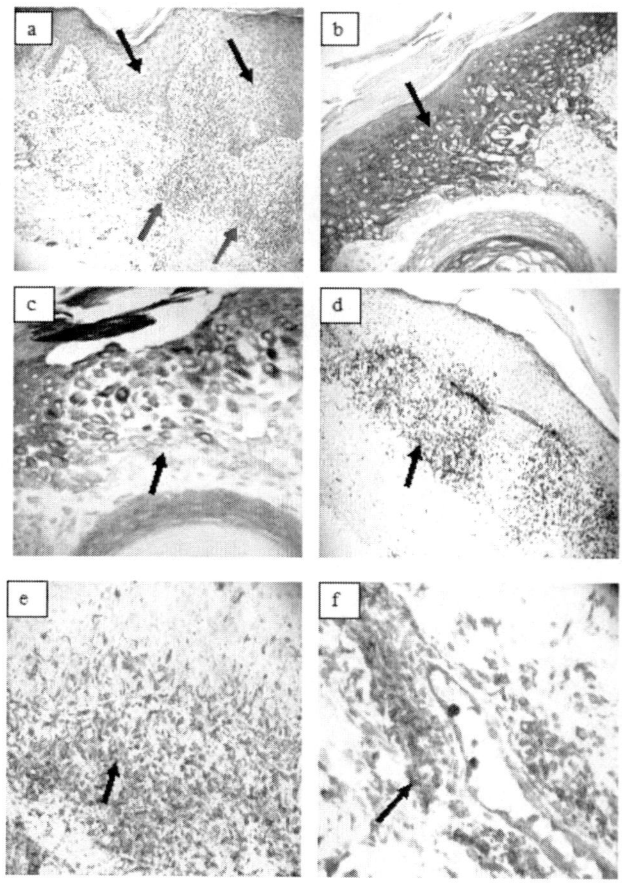

Figure 1. a. H&E staining, showing a focal in situ area of the SCC (black arrows), and the inflammatory infiltrate under the lesion(red arrows) b. Positive IHC staining for AE1/AE3, demonstrating positive staining in the in situ SCC (brown staining; black arrow), as well as on the subjacent infiltrative SCC. c. Positive IHC staining for EMA/CD227 in the in situ SCC (brown staining; black arrow). d. Positive IHC staining for BCL-2 under the in situ SCC (brown staining; black arrow). e and f, Positive IHC staining for HLA-DPDQDR under the in situ SCC, as well as on the perivascular dermal inflammatory infiltrate under the SCC (red staining; black arrows) (200x and 400x, respectively).

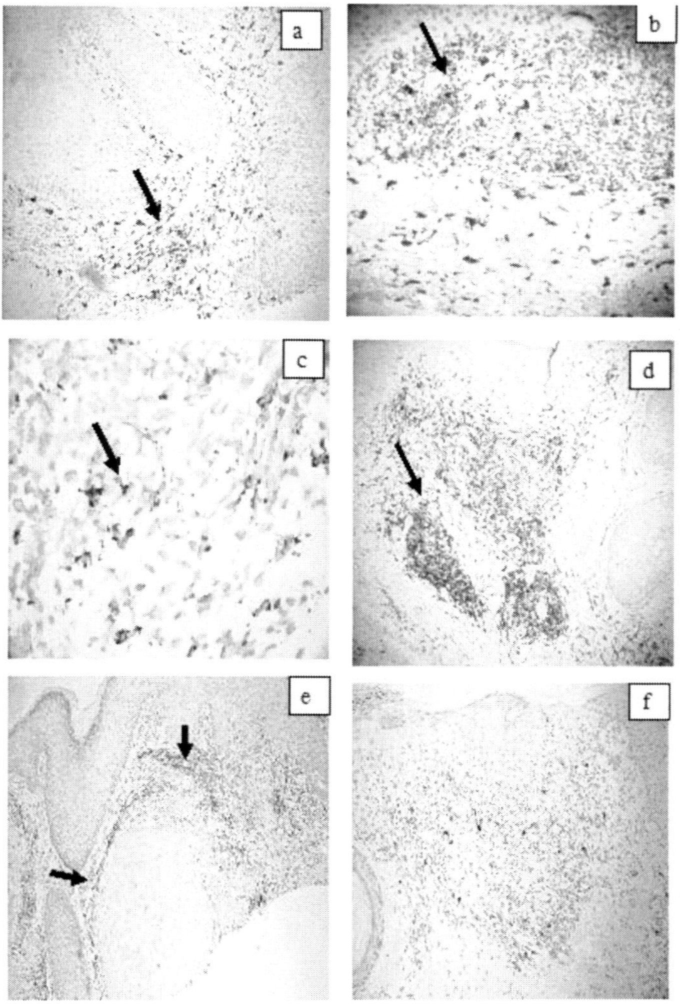

Figure 2. a. Positive IHC staining for CD68, in the inflammatory infiltrate under the SCC (brown staining; black arrow). b. Double IHC stain, showing positive staining for CD68 in brown and Factor XIIIa in red in the dermis and inflammatory infiltrate under the SCC (black arrow). c. Positive staining for HAM56, in the inflammatory infiltrate under the SCC (brown staining; black arrow). d. Positive IHC staining for CD45 in the inflammatory infiltrate under the SCC (brown staining; black arrow). e. Positive IHC staining for CD4, around dermal sides of the SCC (brown staining; black arrows). f. Positive IHC staining for CD57 in the inflammatory infiltrate below the in situ SCC (brown staining).

EMA/CD227 followed a similarly positive pattern of staining as AE1/AE3. CD4, CD8 and CD45 staining was positive around the entire SCC; these markers were also positive inside the tumor. Some positive CD57 cells were seen in the inflammatory infiltrate at tumor base [Figures 1 and 2]. These CD57 positive staining cells displayed somewhat dendritic/neural morphologies. The presence of antigen presenting cells was also noted within the infiltrate, manifested as positive staining for CD68, HAM-56 and Factor XIIIa; these cells were also positive around the tumor in the dermis. HLA-DPDQDR was positive on inflammatory cells inside the tumor, and also around the tumor. BCL-2 was very positive in the tumor, in the epidermis above the tumor, in inflammatory cells around the tumor and around vessels surrounding the tumor [Figures 1 and 2].

Discussion

Pancytokeratin AE1/AE3 and epithelial membrane antigen (EMA/CD227) represent excellent special stains for squamous cell carcinoma, in contradistinction to human epithelial antigen (Ber-EP4), which identifies the basaloid keratinocytes of basal cell carcinoma [6]. In our case, both AE1/AE3 and EMA/CD227 demonstrated diffusely positive, membranous and cytoplasmic staining on the tumor cells.

In regard to the observed positive staining within the immune response infiltrate for HAM56, CD68 and Factor XIIIa, we believe that the immune response is demonstrating strong antigen-presenting cell processing. The process is likely displaying SCC antigens complexed with major histocompatibility complexes (MHCs) to T lymphocytes. The T lymphocytes are then recognizing these complexes utilizing their T cell receptors (TCRs). In the same areas as the antigen presenting cells, we noted a significant population of CD4, CD8 and CD45 positive cells; these cells were present immediately around the SCC, as well as in perivascular areas under the SCC. These combined findings are indicative of a consolidated, directed immune response against the SCC. Other authors have shown also positive staining for CD4, CD8 and CD45 in the context of a human carcinoma immune response [7].

In regards to our positive staining for CD57, the CD57 antigen is a carbohydrate which is also called HNK1 (human natural killer-1) or LEU7. It is expressed as a carbohydrate epitope that contains a sulfoglucuronyl residue, and present in several adhesion molecules of the nervous system as well as on natural killer cells. In anatomic pathology, CD57 IHC is similar to CD56, and utilized in differentiating neuroendocrine, neural and natural killer(NK) cells from other cells. In our CD57 findings, the dermal cells that stained with CD57 exhibited dendritic/neural morphologies. Because the upper dermal neurovascular plexus is present in the area where the positive CD57 staining was observed, we believe we are identifying neural cells with this staining.

Some authors have reported the use of continuous intra-arterial administration of peplomycin (PEP) through a tumor-feeding artery (using an intravascular indwelling catheter) as one of the best treatments for cutaneous SCC in cosmetic areas [8]. Given their results, PEP is useful for the treatment of SCC, and shows immunomodulatory effects on the tumor microenvironment. The authors investigated the immunomodulatory effects of PEP on tumor-infiltrating regulatory T cells, tumor-associated macrophages and CD8 (+)TIA-1(+) cytotoxic T cells in the lesional skin of 5 patients with SCC on the lips [8]. Their data suggest that, in addition to the direct antitumor effects, peplomycin decreased immunosuppressive cells and increased cytotoxic T lymphocytes at the tumor sites; they suggested it might help to maintain a significant immune response against SCC [8].

Other authors investigated putative immunosuppressive cells in SCC and keratoacanthoma (SCCKA), including Tregs and CD163+ macrophages as well as immunomodulatory cells (i.e., IL-27-producing cells) [9]. They also examined the presence of CD3+ Foxp3+ Tregs cells in lesional skin from 10 patients with SCCKA and 18 patients with SCC, and found increased numbers of CD3+ Foxp3+ Tregs in SCC compared with SCCKA. In parallel with Tregs, higher numbers of CD163+ macrophages and MMP-9+ cells were detected (in only the SCCs). In contrast, IL-27-producing cells were increased only in SCCKAs. The authors suggested that the induction of immunosuppressive and immunomodulatory cells differs between SCC and SCCKA [9].

We conclude that, at least in this SCC, there is an active and directed immune response present. Further studies need to be performed to reassess and challenge the concept that most human cancers do not have a significant immune response. In addition, further and larger studies are needed to take therapeutic advantage of such immune responses.

Conflicts of Interest

None.

Funding

Georgia Dermatopathology Associates, Atlanta, Georgia, US.

References

[1] Navarrete-Dechent C, Veness MJ, Droppelmann N, Uribe P. High-risk cutaneous squamous cell carcinoma and the emerging role of sentinel lymph node biopsy: A literature review. *J. Am. Acad. Dermatol.* 2015;73: 127-27.

[2] Abreu Velez AM, Googe PB, Kim J, Howard MS. Markers for sebaceoma show a spectrum of cell cycle regulators, tumor suppressor genes and oncogenes. *North Am. J. Med.*; 2015;7: 275-80.

[3] Abreu Velez AM, Howard MS. Tumor suppressor genes, cell cycle regulatory checkpoints and the skin. *North Am. J. Med.* 2015;7: 176-78.

[4] Abreu Velez AM, Howard MS, Brown VM. A complex immune response in halo nevi correlates with immune reactivity on infiltrated melanocytes, adjacent hair follicles and blood vessels. *Our Derm. Online.* 2014; 5: 391-94.

[5] Abreu Velez AM, Howard MS, Pereyo NG, Delman KA, Mihm MC, Rizzo M. Lymphohistiocytic CD45/CD8 immune response in a case of malignant melanoma, with possible cannibalism. *North Am. J. Med. Sci.;* 2012; 4: 507-09.

[6] Beer TW, Shepherd P, Theaker JM. Ber-EP4 and EMA aid in distinction of basal cell, squamous cell and basosquamous carcinomas of the skin. *Histopathology.* 2000; 37: 218-23.

[7] Rangel R, Rocha L, Ramirez JL, Ibarra MJ, Solorza G, Monroy A, Ramirez MA, Herrera A, Weiss-Steider B. Generation of memory CD4+, CD8+, CD45RO+ and CD16- lymphocytes activated with IL-2, INF-gamma, and TNF-alpha with specific cytotoxicity against autologous cervical cancer cells in a mixed leukocyte-tumour cell culture. *Eur. Cytokine Netw.* 1995;6: 195-02.

[8] Fujimura T, Kambayashi Y, Furudate S, Kakizaki A, Haga T, Hashimoto A, et al. Immunomodulatory effects of peplomycin on immunosuppressive and cytotoxic cells in the lesional skin of cutaneous squamous cell carcinoma. *Dermatology. 2015*;230: 250-55.

[9] Kambayashi Y, Fujimura T, Aiba S. Comparison of immunosuppressive and immunomodulatory cells in keratoacanthoma and cutaneous squamous cell carcinoma. *Acta Derm. Venereol.* 2013;93: 663-68.

In: Inflammatory Markers, Oncogenes … ISBN: 978-1-63484-303-4
Editor: Ana Maria Abreu Velez

Chapter 11

DOUBLE COLOR IMMUNOHISTOCHEMISTRY ANALYSIS OF THE IMMUNE RESPONSE, ANGIOLYMPHATIC INVASION AND TUMOR MITOTIC RATE IN A SUPERFICIAL SPREADING MALIGNANT MELANOMA

Ana Maria Abreu Velez[1,*], MD, PhD, E. D. DeLoach[2], MD, FACS and Michael S. Howard[1], MD

[1]Georgia Dermatopathology Associates, Atlanta, Georgia, US
[2]Savannah Plastic Surgery Associates, Savannah, Georgia, US

ABSTRACT

Context: In the medical literature, the *in situ* malignant melanoma immune response has been often described as unproductive. *Case report:* A 44 year old male presented with a slowly growing and changing, asymmetric flat patch of hyperpigmented skin on the left breast. A lesional punch biopsy was taken to study hematoxylin and eosin (H&E)

* Corresponding author: Ana Maria Abreu Velez, MD, PhD, Georgia Dermatopathology Associates, 1534 North Decatur Road., NE; Suite 206; Atlanta, Georgia 30307-1000 USA. E-mail: abreuvelez@yahoo.com, Telephone: (404) 371-0077, Toll Free: (877) 371-0027, Fax: (404) 371-1900.

histologic features, as well as possible immunohistochemistry (IHC) analysis. The H&E review demonstrated an atypical melanocytic proliferation, with single cells, and nests located along the dermal/epidermal junction. Focally, well developed epidermal pagetoid permeation of neoplastic cells was also identified. Atypical melanocytes also invaded the dermis as single cells. The tumor cells displayed variable cytologic atypia. IHC staining demonstrated diffusely positive staining on the tumor cells with S-100 and Mart-1/Melan A/CD63. Focal staining was noted within the tumor for CD8 and CD45. A few CD20 positive lymphocytes were seen in some parts of the tumor. Galectin-3 was very positive throughout most of the tumor. HLA-DP, DQ, DR antigen, Factor XIIIa and CD68 demonstrated positive staining on cells within the tumor. The tumor cell proliferation rate was confirmed utilizing Ki-67 staining. Although the H&E sections failed to demonstrate tumor cell angiolymphatic invasion, double IHC staining confirmed metastatic tumor cells within dermal blood vessels via CD31, CD34, D2-40 and melanoma specific markers. *Conclusion:* The advantages of double color IHC staining in malignant melanoma workups include tissue conservation, confirmation of angiolymphatic invasion and studying the melanoma immune response. Selected dermatopathology laboratories routinely utilize double IHC staining. Using this technique, we were able to accomplish these goals in our workup.

Keywords: superficial spreading malignant melanoma, *in situ* immune response, double immunohistochemistry staining, Ki-67, Galectin-3, CD8, CD25, CD45, CD68, Factor XIIIa

ABBREVIATIONS

H&E	Hematoxylin and eosin
IHC	immunohistochemistry
BMZ	basement membrane zone
SSM	superficial spreading melanoma
SLN	sentinel lymph node

INTRODUCTION

Superficial spreading malignant melanoma (SSM) is the most common subtype of melanoma (it accounts for approximately 70% of melanomas) [1-

3]. Melanoma represents a potentially fatal skin cancer, that arises from melanocytes [1-3]. Superficial spreading melanoma is a form of melanoma in which the malignant cells tend to stay confined to the epidermis (the "*in-situ*" phase) for a prolonged period [1-3]. Initially, superficial spreading melanoma grows horizontally within the epidermis and along the basement membrane zone [BMZ] of the skin; this growth begins the radial growth phase. The lesions often present clinically as slowly enlarging, flat pigmented macules or plaques with inconsistently defined borders and color variation. Prognostic factors and indications for sentinel lymph node (SLN) biopsies are important to identify in SSM [1-3]. A subset of SSMs become invasive, ie, the melanoma cells cross the BMZ and enter the dermis; these cells then may initiate a vertical growth phase tumor [1-3]. Although more common in fair skinned individuals (Fitzpatrick Phototypes 1 and 2), SSM may also occur in those who tan easily (Phototype 3). SSM is uncommon in brown or black skin (Phototypes 4-6). Superficial spreading melanoma presents equally seen in both sexes, and is less common before the age of 40 [1-3]. Dermatoscopy can help to clinically detect these malignancies. The main risk factors for SSM include increasing age, a personal history of previous melanoma or nonmelanoma skin cancer, multiple melanocytic nevi, and a significant family history of melanoma, especially with 2 or more first degree relatives affected.

CASE REPORT

A 44 year old male white male presented to the plastic surgeon's office with several skin lesions about which he was concerned. The patient was referred by his primary care physician, and presented with a patch of hyperpigmented skin on the left breast. On clinical examination, the lesion demonstrated some asymmetry, border irregularity and color variation. The lesional skin was punch biopsied, and analyzed utilizing hematoxylin and eosin (H&E) staining, as well as by immunohistochemistry (IHC). After the skin biopsy results were received, a conservative excision of an invasive malignant melanoma of the left breast was performed. To cover the surgical defect, a 15 cm length by 4.5 cm width flap repair was made.

Materials and Methods

H&E and Immunohistochemistry (IHC): We performed out H&E staining as previously described [4-7]. In our IHC testing, we utilized a dual endogenous peroxidase blockage, with the addition of a Dako Envision dual link (to assist in chromogen attachment). We then applied the chromogen 3,3-diaminobenzidine (DAB), and counterstained with hematoxylin. The samples were run in a Dako Autostainer Universal Staining System. Positive and negative controls were consistently performed. Our staining was performed as previously described [4-7]. We performed IHC utilizing multiple monoclonal and polyclonal antibodies from Dako (Carpinteria, California, USA). We utilized mouse anti-human monoclonal mouse HLA-DP, DQ, DR antigen, clone CR3/43; S-100; Mart-1/Melan A/CD63; melanoma associated antigen(PNL2); CD4; CD8, Clone C8/144B; Clone DO-7; CD20, Clone L26; CD25; CD31/PECAM; CD34; anti-human CD45/Leukcocyte Common Antigen, Clone 2B11 + PD7/26; CD68; podoplanin/D2-40; Factor XIIIa; PPG9.5; Galectin 3 and Ki-67.

IHC double staining: Our IHC double stains were performed utilizing a Leica (Buffalo Grove, Illinois, USA) double staining system. Specifically, for primary staining we utilized a Bond Max platform autostainer with bond polymer refined red detection DS9390, an alkaline phosphatase linker polymer and a fast red chromogen (red staining). For our secondary staining, we utilized bond polymer refined detection DS9800, a horseradish peroxidase linker polymer and a DAB chromogen (brown staining). Positive and negative controls were consistently performed, as previously reported [4-7]. The following antibodies were utilized from Leica/Novocastra: monoclonal mouse anti-human polyclonal rabbit anti-human CD3, monoclonal mouse anti-human CD20 and anti-human glial fibrillary acidic protein (GFAP).

Results

Microscopic H&E results: Examination of the H&E tissue sections demonstrated an atypical melanocytic proliferation. Specifically, atypical melanocytes were present as single cells, runs of cells, and nests located along the dermal/epidermal junction (basement membrane zone; BMZ). In addition,

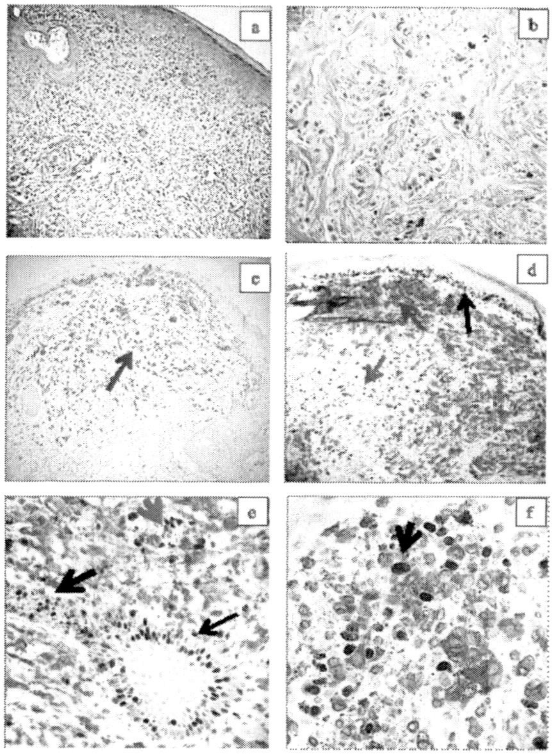

Figure 1. Histologic features and tumoral proliferation rate. 1. a and b, H&E staining at 100 and 400x respectively, showing melanoma cells descending from the junctional zone, and infiltrating the dermis. c. S-100 IHC staining highlights that the malignant melanocytes infiltrating the dermis (brown staining; red arrow). d. Double IHC staining, utilizing using Ki-67 (dark brown staining) showing active cellular proliferation, and colocalizing with melanoma cells at the junctional zone stained with Mart-1/Melan A/CD63(red staining); (black arrow). Please note that below in the dermis, only scattered Ki-67 staining is seen within groups of melanoma cells (blue arrow). Please also note that there are some areas free of tumor in the dermis, where non-melanoma cells demonstrate positive Ki-67 staining (green arrow); in these areas, we later confirmed the presence of multiple immune system cells. In e, the stains are similar to d, and we highlight a hair follicle BMZ strongly expressing Ki-67 (black arrows). Adjacent dermal areas show combined positive staining of melanoma cells and Ki-67 (green arrow). f. Similar staining as in e; showing that immediately subjacent to the epidermis, only a few malignant melanocytes are also positive for Ki-67 (black arrow).

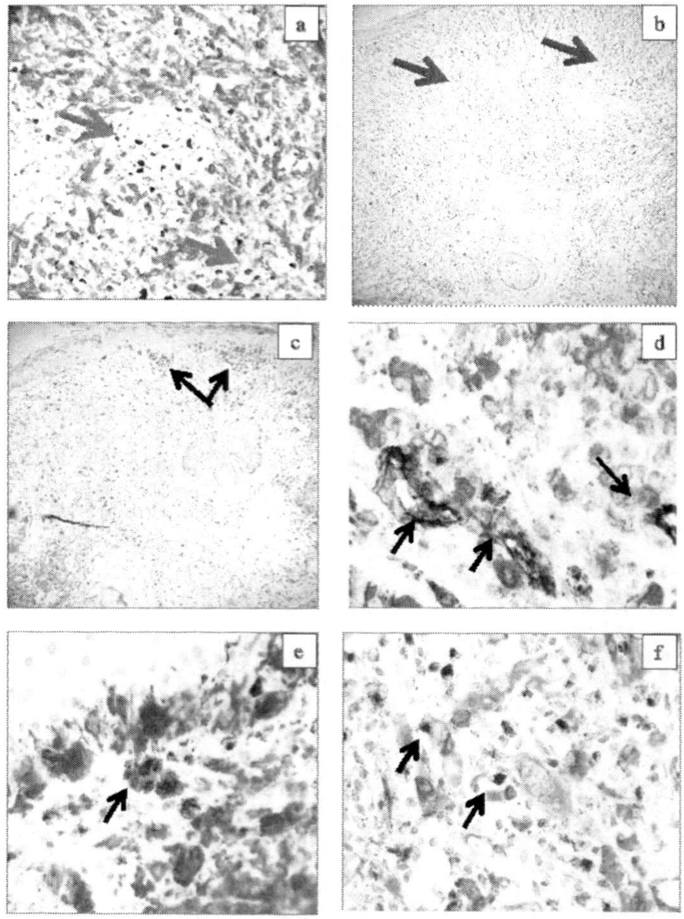

Figure 2. a. Double staining IHC, demonstrating Mart-1/Melan A/CD63 in red, and Ki-67 in brown. We highlight dermal area free of invasive malignant melanocytes, where other cells are highly proliferative per Ki-67 staining (brown staining; green arrows). b. Double staining IHC, with Galectin-3 in brown and CD25 in red. These markers colocalize within the tumor (blue arrows) (40x). In c, similar to b, but shows areas where Galactin-3 expression is strongly concentrated immediately subjacent to the BMZ (brown staining; black arrows). d. Double staining IHC, using Mart-1/Melan A/CD63 (in red) and D2-40/podoplanin (in brown), and demonstrating that melanoma cells are in contact with and/or invading dermal lymphatic vessels (black arrows) (400x). e. Double staining IHC, showing Mart-1/Melan A/CD63 in red and CD68 in brown. Please note that a very large, CD68 positive cell under the BMZ seems to have phagocytosed all or portions of a melanoma cell (black arrow) (400x). f. Same stain as in e, but this shows how the CD68 positive cells seem to be "guarding and surrounding" the melanoma cells(black arrows) (40X).

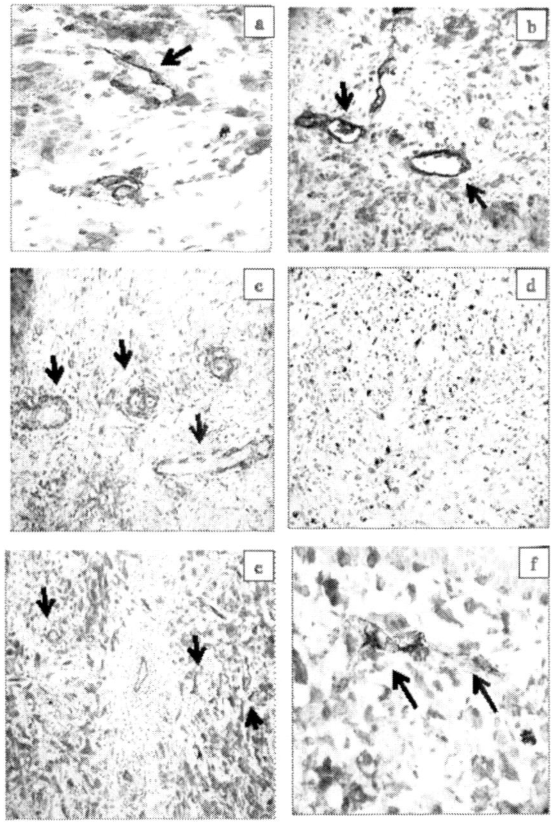

Figure 3. Metastases of melanoma cells. a. Double staining IHC, showing CD34 on dermal blood vessel endothelial cells in brown and Mart-1/Melan A/CD63 in red; we highlight an approach of malignant melanocytes to the edges of a blood vessel(black arrow) (200x). b. Double staining IHC, showing staining of dermal lymphatic endothelial cells with D2-40/podoplanin in brown, and malignant melanocytes with Mart-1/Melan A/CD63 in red. Note the malignant melanocytes approaching the lymphatic vessels (black arrows) (200x). c. Single staining IHC staining for CD45 in red, showing diffusely positive dermal staining, accentuated around vessels (black arrows), and including vessels supplying an eccrine sweat gland(blue arrow) (100x). d. Double staining IHC, showing some colocalization of CD68 (brown staining), and Factor XIIIa (red staining), within the tumor (200X). e. Metastases were detected in small dermal blood vessels by using double IHC staining. Melanoma cells are stained with Mart-1/Melan A/CD63 (red staining), and blood vessel endothelial cells with CD31/PECAM(brown staining)(black arrows) (100x). f. Double IHC staining, presenting a proximity between the melanoma cells stained with Mart-1/Melan A/CD63 (red staining), and lymphatic endothelial cells stained with D2-40/podoplanin(brown staining) (black arrow).

atypical melanocytes invaded the papillary dermis as single cells. Focally, well developed, epidermal pagetoid permeation of neoplastic cells was also identified. Individual atypical melanocytes were of small to large size, and displayed epithelioid morphology; these cells displayed variable cytologic atypia. The atypical melanocytes contained round to oval nuclei with fine, dispersed chromatin and small, eosinophilic nucleoli. Occasional intranuclear inclusions are noted within the neoplastic melanocytes. Moderate amounts of eosinophilic cytoplasm are present within these cells (see Figure 1).

Lesional melanocytic mitotic figures are rare, quantified at 0-1 per high powered (400x) microscopic field. A mild host inflammatory response was noted, with small numbers of tumor infiltrating lymphocytes observed; however, no areas of frank histologic regression were seen. No vascular space invasion, perineural invasion, or lymphatic invasion was identified using H&E staining. No tumoral ulceration or satellitosis was appreciated. The neoplastic process contacted the lateral punch biopsy specimen borders in the sections examined.

IHC results: Diffusely positive, membranous and cytoplasmic staining was noted on the tumor cells on review of the S-100, Mart-1/Melan A/CD63 and PNL2 special stains. The tumor staining was concentrated along the basement membrane zone of the skin.

The stains for S-100 and Mart-1/Melan A/CD63 were not evenly distributed throughout the tumor [see Figures 1 through 6]. Galectin-3 was very positive in areas of the BMZ where tumor cells were also present [see Figure 3]. Galectin-3 positive cells demonstrated colocalization with CD25 positive cells [see Figure 2]. The area positivity and stain density of Galectin-3 and CD25 overlapped, but their expression varied throughout the tumor.

Our staining for CD4 positive cells was negative within the tumor. Our CD20 staining was positive on a few cells, localized in only one area of the tumor [see Figure 4]. Melanoma cells unevenly expressed Ki-67. The Ki-67 positive tumor cells were also present in higher numbers along the dermal/epidermal junction, and within BMZ areas of hair follicular units. In addition, endothelial cell areas in several dermal vessels expressed Ki-67 colocalizing with D2-40/podoplanin, von Willembrand factor and CD34 [see Figures 2 and 3].

Although no definitive angiolymphatic invasion was noted on H&E review, microscopic metastases were confirmed via IHC, specifically via double IHC staining. The double staining demonstrated metastases in several small dermal vessels by colocalization of S-100 and Mart-1/Melan A/CD63 with CD34, D2-40/podoplanin and von Willembrand factor [see Figure 3].

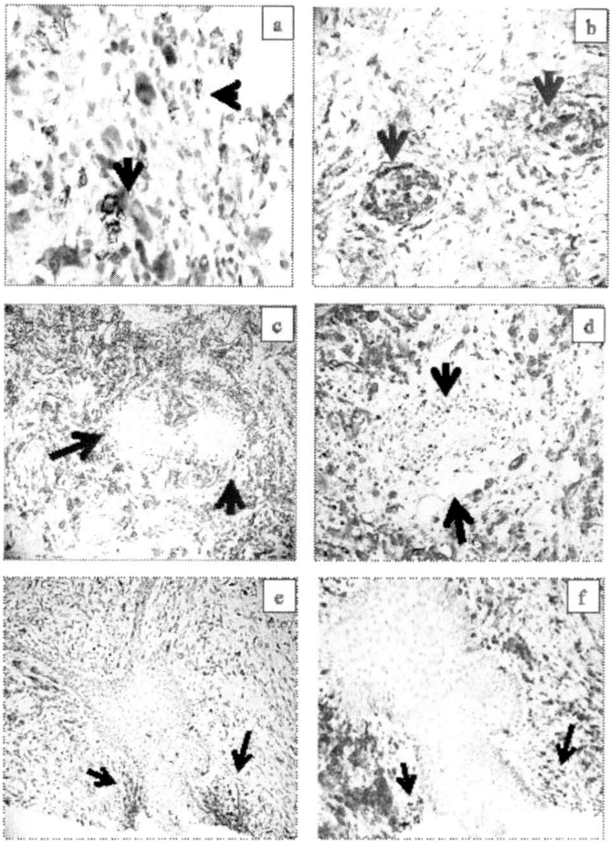

Figure 4. The immune response and melanoma cells. In a, a double staining IHC, using S-100(red staining) and CD20 (brown staining). Please note than the melanoma cells are less common in areas where the CD20 staining is positive (black arrows), indicating some type of immunologic control exerted by B lymphocytes over the melanoma cells. In b, using again double IHC staining, we note colocalization of CD8 (brown staining) around the vessels (blue arrows); these cells represent a subset of CD45 positive cells (red staining). c. Note that Mart-1/Melan A/CD63 positive staining (brown staining) is decreased around selected dermal vessels where the immune cells were located in b (blue arrows). d. Double staining IHC, showing positive CD68 cells (brown staining; black arrows), around dermal vessels. Again, note that Mart-1/Melan A/CD63 positive melanoma cells (red staining) are uncommon in areas where the antigen presenting cells predominate. e Another example, showing cluster areas around a hair follicle where CD45 positive cells are present(red staining; black arrows). CD8 cells are highlighted as well (brown staining). f. Double staining IHC, showing the same cluster areas as in e, but the staining in this case is against CD68(brown staining) and Mart-1/Melan A/CD63(red staining)(black arrows).

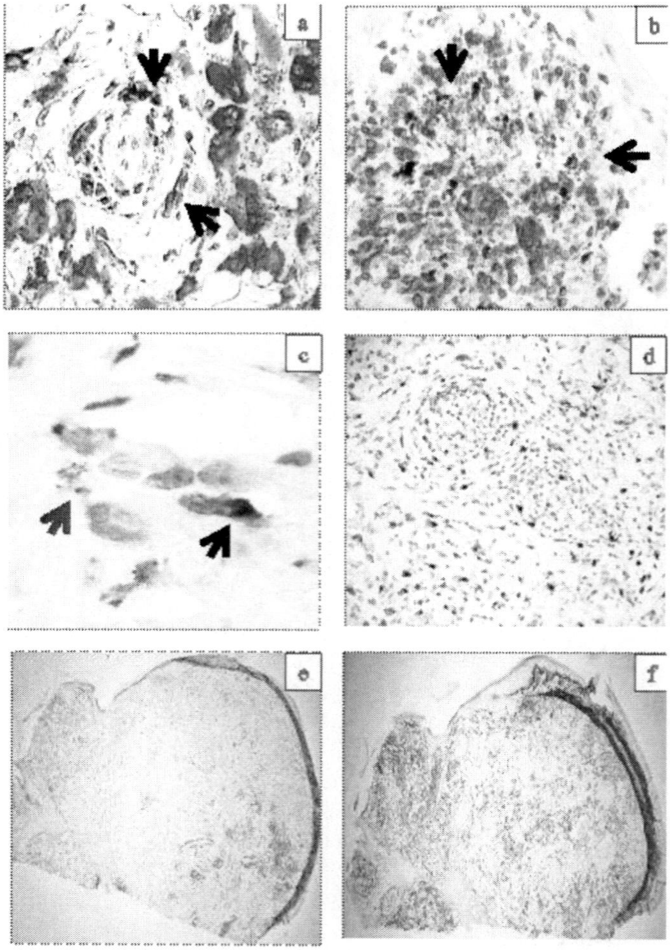

Figure 5. Melanoma immune response. a. Double staining IHC, showing positive CD68 cells (brown staining; black arrows) colocalizing with Factor XIIIa staining (red staining). b. Double staining IHC, showing positive CD68 cells (brown staining) infiltrating and encircling melanoma cells staining positive Melan A in red (black arrows)(200x). c. Double staining IHC shows that some dermal immune response cells (near the melanoma) colocalized the CD68 marker (brown staining) with Factor XIIIa (red staining)(black arrow); however, this colocalization was not present other immune response cells in the immediate area(red arrow) (100x).d. Double staining IHC, with CD68 (brown staining) and Factor XIIIa (red staining) infiltrating melanoma cells around dermal vessels. e. Double IHC staining with CD8 (brown staining) and CD45 (red staining)(40x). f. Single staining IHC, highlighting CD8 positive staining cells within the tumor (40x).

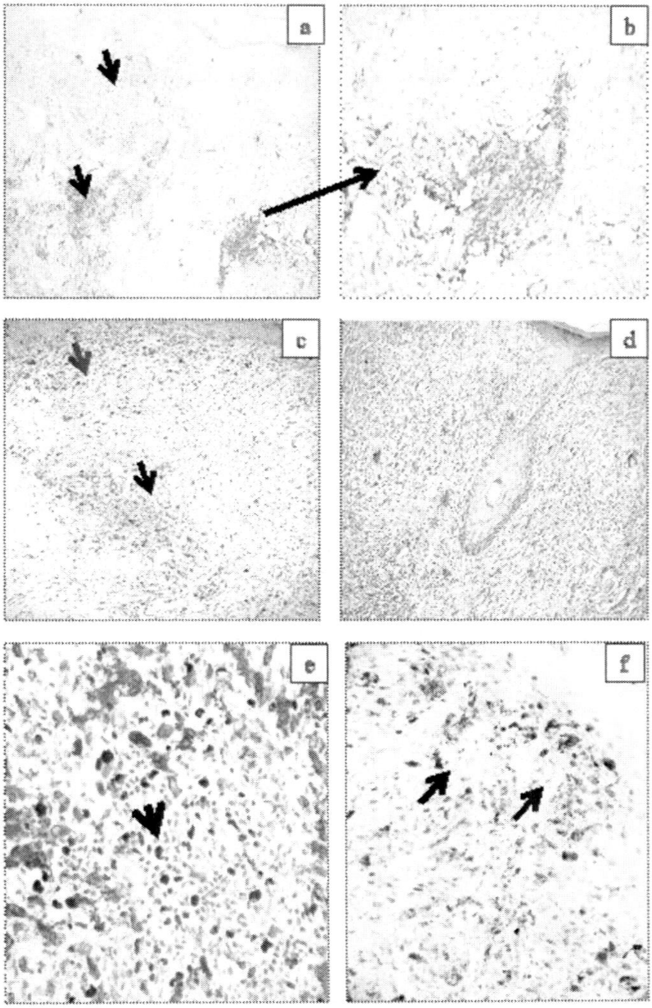

Figure 6. a and b. Double staining IHC, using CD4 (largely negative) (brown staining) and HLA-DP,DQ,DR antigen (red staining) positive in patchy areas of the tumor (black arrows). In b, higher magnification of a (black arrow). c. Double staining IHC, with Galectin 3 showing some clustered areas below the BMZ (brown staining; red arrow), and CD25 (red staining) showing patchy reactivity (black arrow) (100x). d. H&E staining, shows the patchy dermal presentation of the melanoma cells (100x). e. Double staining IHC, showing positive staining for Ki-67 (brown staining; black arrow); the staining is present in areas of T lymphocyte and/or antigen presenting cells close to dermal vessels, but not much is present infiltrating the melanoma cells, marked by Melan A (red staining). f. Double staining IHC, showing positive staining with CD8 (brown staining) and CD45 (red staining) (black arrows) (200x).

CD8 was positive in several areas of the tumor, but no particular pattern of positivity was appreciated. The CD8 positive cells accumulated in the areas along the BMZ confirmed as tumoral areas via melanoma markers. Positive staining for CD45 stain was also identified in multiple dermal areas containing positive staining for melanoma cells. A similar positive staining pattern was seen with CD68, especially around several large dermal vessels in the vicinity of tumor cells.

Moreover, CD68 positive cells were noted in the majority of the tumor area, in patterns that seemed to be inversely related to the presence of melanoma cells. For example, in several areas where the strongest CD68 staining was noted, Mart-1/Melan A/CD63 positive tumor cells were relatively sparse. In contrast, our CD8 and CD68 staining often directly correlated in tumor cell areas.

Finally, HLA DP, DQ, DR antigen demonstrated positive staining, especially throughout the upper dermal plexus of neurovascular structures [see Figure 6]. HLA-DP, DQ, DR antigen was also positive around peritumoral area neovascular structures in the dermis [see Figure 6].

Discussion

Superficial spreading melanoma often presents clinically as a slowly growing and changing, flat patch of hyperpigmented skin [1-3]. Initially, it frequently resembles a benign nevus or dysplastic nevus. Like other flat forms of melanoma, it can be often recognized by the ABCDE parameters: Asymmetry, Border irregularity, Color variation, Diameter and Evolution (ABCDE) [1-3]. The clinical characteristics of SSM include: 1) a larger size than most benign nevi (>6 mm and often 1-2 centimeters in diameter); 2) irregular shape; 3) variable pigmentation including light brown, dark brown, black, blue, grey, pink and red colors; and 4) a smooth surface at first, later becoming thicker with an irregular surface that may be dry or warty [1-3]. Intermittent sun exposure seems to play a major etiologic role in SSM, which has demonstrated increasing incidence over recent decades [3].

In our case, we found that melanoma cells confirmed on H&E review and via the S-100 and Mart-1/Melan A/CD63 stains were present in interesting patterns inside the tumor. These two markers were particularly positive in several areas of the basement membrane zone where the melanoma had originated. In contradistinction, these markers were less positive on some dermal tumor cells. Ki-67 was also very positive in the BMZ area, possibly indicating a high proliferation rate on these transformed malignant cells. The significance of these findings is not known.

Relative to melanoma and the *in situ* immune response, it is currently accepted that the human immune response in melanoma is not largely effective [8]. We searched the entire PubMed online data base; to our surprise, not many well controlled studies evaluating the *in situ* immune response in melanoma were found. In contrast, we found that many manuscripts evaluated attempts to elicit a melanoma immune response *in vitro*, via animal and human studies. Many therapies are in development to overcome melanoma immune response anergy, including 1) addressing immune checkpoint blockade, and 2) tumor radiation therapy as a strategy to perform an *in situ* immunization; such a strategy would produce "immunogenic cell death," and elicit a local immune response. Other therapeutic trials include 3) the use of topical immune response modifiers such as imiquimod and resiquimod [9-13].

Not all of the proliferating cells we identified with Ki-67 staining are melanoma cells. Thus, other cells are proliferating around the melanoma; these cells are likely involved in the melanoma immune response. When chemotherapy is given to patients with melanoma, the chemotherapy acts against all cells that exhibit a high proliferative rate. In our case, we found positive staining on putative immune response cells and vascular markers colocalizing with our Ki-67 staining. Again, if chemotherapy is utilized to address melanoma, any proliferating *in situ* immune cells will also be affected, slowing the "natural immune response." Finally, the observed positivity of our Ki-67 in hair follicle cells is interpreted as related to the normal anagen phase of hair growth.

In regard to the positive Galectin-3 staining in our case, this protein has been shown to be involved in multiple biological processes, including cell adhesion, cell activation, chemoattraction, inflammation, cell growth, cancer genesis, cell cycle regulation and apoptosis [14-17]. Overexpression and changes in the intercellular localization of Galectin-3 are commonly seen in cancerous conditions. We found one study showing *in situ* localization of Galectin-3 with melanoma cells, as we observed in our case [17]. These findings suggest the possibility of reviewing large numbers of melanomas for Galectin-3 expression, trying to find patterns of prognostic and/or therapeutic value.

As we observed in this case, lymphocytic and plasma cell infiltration around a malignant tumor probably represents an immunologic response of the host directed against the neoplasm. Using double IHC staining detecting simultaneous colocalization of melanoma cells and CD20, we noted that the melanoma cells were present in decreased numbers in areas of CD20 expression. Thus, the staining pattern suggests a possible immunologic control in these areas, exerted over the melanoma cells. Importantly, minimal and focal CD20 positivity was seen throughout the melanoma.

The CD8 and CD45 positive IHC staining also exhibited interesting patterns inside and around the SSM. Inside the SSM, it was difficult for us to determine any specific correlation of patterns between the melanoma cells and the immune response cells. However, dual CD8 and CD45 positive immune response cells seemed to be concentrated around peritumoral dermal vessels (both lymphatics and blood vessels). We also noted antigen presenting cells, positively identified via CD68 and Factor XIIIa, to be concentrated in these same sites. Thus, we could identify a robust and biphasic cellular immune response present in peritumoral, tumor-free areas around these dermal vessels.

The immune response in this case of SMM was also manifested via positive staining for CD25. The CD25 antigen is the alpha chain of the IL-2 receptor. The interleukin-2 receptor (IL-2R) is a heterotrimeric protein expressed on the surface of specific immune system cells, including lymphocytes. It is a type I transmembrane protein present on activated B and T lymphocytes, some thymocytes, myeloid precursors, and oligodendrocytes. CD25 associates with CD122 to form a heterodimer, which can then serve as a high-affinity receptor for IL-2. Since we found a strong presence of CD25 positive T lymphocytes in the SSM, it is plausible to suggest that these cells are participating in tumor specific activation of the host immune system. The presence of CD25 positive cells in cutaneous melanoma has also been previously described by others [19] The full role of CD25 in the development of T cell immunologic memory needs further study. However, it is possible that CD25 positive T lymphocytes expand the number and function of antigen-selected clones, and that these clones play a key role in enduring cell-mediated immunity in melanoma.

In general, it is accepted that tumor cell proliferation is positively correlated with the progression of melanoma. Accordingly, the proliferation index of H&E-stained thin melanomas was recently included in the staging system of the American Joint Committee on Cancer with other parameters [19]. Besides Ki-67, other emerging proliferation markers such as phosphohistone H3, minichromosome maintenance protein 4 and mitosin have been utilized as proliferative markers for melanoma cells [20]. Of interest, we noted that positive Ki-67 staining colocalized with immune cells including T lymphocytes, antigen presenting cells and HLA-DP, DQ, DR positive cells.

Thus, we suggest that these immune response cells are indeed proliferating, indicating an active cellular immune response.

Several melanoma-associated antigens recognized by T cells have been identified, including multiple HLA class I- and class II-restricted peptides. These antigens have then been classified as tumor-associated testis-specific antigens, melanocyte differentiation antigens, and mutated or aberrantly expressed antigens [21]. These proteins give rise to several antigenic peptides. The number of known melanoma-associated peptides that can induce killing by cytotoxic T-lymphocytes exceeds 30, and is increasing. Consistent with these findings, clinical data indicate that the immune system is essential in control of tumor growth. Further, immunomodulatory therapies have accomplished complete or partial tumor regression in a number of patients.

The metastasis of melanoma via dermal vessels was not appreciated on H&E review. However, utilizing double staining IHC, we demonstrated metastases in small vessels using melanoma markers such as S-100 and Mart-1/Melan A/CD63 colocalizing with positive vascular staining for von Willembrand factor, CD34 and D2-40/podoplanin. Here, the advantage of simultaneous, double color IHC staining was confirmed. We also utilized the neural marker PPG.9.5; however, due to the punctate nature of its positive staining and the thin anatomy of dermal nerves, we were not able to confirm perineural SSM metastases via IHC double staining. The double staining IHC technique thus supersedes conventional (single color) IHC power of analysis when investigating primary melanoma and associated metastases [22].

Conclusion

The primary tumor cells, metastasizing cells, immune system response cells and proliferation markers were unevenly observed within the tumor. These findings demonstrate the oncologic concept of a "tumor inside the tumor." How can we know if an *in situ* immune response to melanoma is a clinically effective response? As stated previously, the immune system response in most melanomas has been interpreted as inadequate to control tumor growth and metastases. Double staining IHC techniques allow a more comprehensive study of the melanoma *in situ* immune response. Additional power of analysis may be attained via sequential sections taken through a melanoma, with the double staining IHC technique then applied to progressively deeper areas within a single tumor.

ACKNOWLEDGMENTS

Jonathan S. Jones, HT(ASCP) at Georgia Dermatopathology Associates provided excellent technical assistance.

Conflicts of Interest

None.

Funding

Georgia Dermatopathology Associates, Atlanta, Georgia, US.

REFERENCES

[1] Debarbieux S, Thomas L; Groupe imagerie cutanée non invasive de la Société française de dermatologie. Superficial spreading melanoma. *Ann. Dermatol. Venereol.* 2015;142:66-69.

[2] Egger ME, Stepp LO, Callender GG, Quillo AR, Martin RC 2nd, Scoggins CR, et al. Outcomes and prognostic factors in superficial spreading melanoma. *Am. J. Surg.* 2013;206:861-67.

[3] Micu E, Baturaite Z, Juzeniene A, Bruland ØS, Moan JE. Superficial-spreading and nodular melanomas in Norway: a comparison by body site distribution and latitude gradients. *Melanoma Res.* 2012;22:460-65.

[4] Abreu Velez AM, Howard MS, Pereyo NG, Delman KA, Mihm MC, Rizzo M. Lymphohistiocytic CD45/CD8 immune response in a case of malignant melanoma, with possible cannibalism. *North Am. J. Med. Sci.* 2012. 4: 507-09.

[5] Abreu Velez AM, Howard MS. Immune reactivity in psoriatic Munro-Saboureau microabscesses, stratum corneum and blood vessels. *North Am J Med Sci.* 2012. 4:257-65.

[6] Abreu Velez AM, Howard MS. HAM56 and CD68 antigen presenting cells surrounding a sarcoidal granulomatous tattoo. DeJoseph LM. *North Am J Med Sci.* 2011; 3: 475-77.

[7] Abreu Velez AM, Brown VM, Howard MS. An inflamed trichilemmal (pilar) cyst: Not so simple? *North Am. J. Med. Sci.* 2011; 3: 431-34.

[8] Janeway CA Jr, Travers P, Walport M, et al. Immunobiology: The Immune System in Health and Disease. 5th edition. New York: Garland Science; 2001.

[9] Makkouk A, Joshi VB, Wongrakpanich A, Lemke CD, Gross BP, Salem AK, Weiner GJ. Biodegradable microparticles loaded with doxorubicin and CpG ODN for in situ immunization against cancer. *AAPS J.* 2015;17:184-93.

[10] Marabelle A, Filatenkov A, Sagiv-Barfi I, Kohrt H. Radiotherapy and toll-like receptor agonists. *Semin. Radiat. Oncol.* 2015;25:34-39.

[11] Liu Y, Xiao L, Joo KI, Hu B, Fang J, Wang P. In situ modulation of dendritic cells by injectable thermosensitive hydrogels for cancer vaccines in mice. *Biomacromolecules.* 2014 13;3836-45.

[12] Li X, Naylor MF, Le H, Nordquist RE, Teague TK, Howard CA, Murray C, Chen WR. Clinical effects of in situ photoimmunotherapy on late-stage melanoma patients: a preliminary study. *Cancer Biol. Ther.* 2010;10:1081-87.

[13] Woodmansee C, Pillow J, Skinner RB Jr. The role of topical immune response modifiers in skin cancer. *Drugs.* 2006;66:1657-64.

[14] Newlaczyl A, Yu L. "Galectin-3--a jack-of-all-trades in cancer." *Cancer Letters.* 2011; 313: 123–28.

[15] Henderson N, Sethi T. "The regulation of inflammation by galectin-3." *Immunological Reviews.* 2009; 230: 160–61.

[16] Prieto VG, Mourad-Zeidan AA, Melnikova V, Johnson MM, Lopez A, Diwan AH, et al. Galectin-3 expression is associated with tumor progression and pattern of sun exposure in melanoma. *Clin. Cancer Res.* 2006;12:6709-15.

[17] Zubieta MR, Furman D, Barrio M, Bravo AI, Domenichini E, Mordoh J. Galectin-3 expression correlates with apoptosis of tumor-associated lymphocytes in human melanoma biopsies. *Am. J. Pathol.* 2006;168:1666-75.

[18] 18 Kernohan NM, Sewell HF.Interleukin-2 receptor expression in benign and malignant melanocytic skin lesions. *J. Pathol.* 1989;157:315-19.

[19] Nielsen PS, Riber-Hansen R, Jensen TO, Schmidt H, Steiniche T. Proliferation indices of phosphohistone H3 and Ki67: strong prognostic markers in a consecutive cohort with stage I/II melanoma. *Mod. Pathol.* 2013;26:404-13.

[20] Ladstein RG, Bachmann IM, Straume O, Akslen LA. Ki-67 expression is superior to mitotic count and novel proliferation markers PHH3, MCM4 and mitosin as a prognostic factor in thick cutaneous melanoma. *BMC Cancer*. 2010;10:140.

[21] Thor Straten P, Becker JC, Guldberg P, Zeuthen J. In situ T cells in melanoma. *Cancer Immunol Immunother*. 1999;48:386-95.

[22] Storr SJ, Safuan S, Mitra A, Elliott F, Walker C, Vasko MJ, Ho B, Cook M, Mohammed RA, Patel PM, Ellis IO, Newton-Bishop JA, Martin SG. Objective assessment of blood and lymphatic vessel invasion and association with macrophage infiltration in cutaneous melanoma. *Mod. Pathol.* 2012;25:493-94.

In: Inflammatory Markers, Oncogenes … ISBN: 978-1-63484-303-4
Editor: Ana Maria Abreu Velez

Chapter 12

AGGRESSIVE NODULAR BASAL CELL CARCINOMA WITH EXPRESSION OF PROLIFERATING CELL NUCLEAR ANTIGEN AND B-CELL LYMPHOMA 2 GENE

Ana Maria Abreu Velez[1,*], MD PhD, Rick Lockhart[2], MD and Michael S. Howard[1], MD
[1]Georgia Dermatopathology Associates, Atlanta, Georgia, US
[2]Middle Georgia Ear, Nose and Throat Surgery Center, Milledgeville, Georgia, US

ABSTRACT

Context: The distinction between basal cell carcinoma (BCC) and other tumors is classically made on the basis of defined histological criteria, with the possible addition of immunohistochemistry staining (IHC).

Case report: A 57 year old male presented with a large mass on his left cheek. A lesional punch biopsy was taken to review hematoxylin and

* Corresponding author: Ana Maria Abreu Velez, MD, PhD, Georgia Dermatopathology Associates, 1534 North Decatur Road., NE; Suite 206; Atlanta, Georgia 30307-1000 USA. E-mail: abreuvelez@yahoo.com, Telephone: (404) 371-0077, Toll Free: (877) 371-0027, Fax: (404) 371-1900.

eosin (H&E) histologic features, as well as for possible immunohistochemistry (IHC) analysis.

Results: The H&E review demonstrated a malignant neoplasm comprised of focal aggregates of basaloid keratinocytes with hyperchromatic nuclei and minimal cytoplasm. Palisading of peripheral nuclei within the basaloid aggregates was also noted. IHC staining confirmed a diagnosis of BCC, with focal squamous differentiation. BCL-2 and PCNA were positive in the palisaded areas of the tumor. Vimentin was positive in the central, necrotic parts of the tumor. Cox-2 was positive in only a few, focal areas of the tumor.

Conclusion: In this BCC, other stains beyond Ber-Ep4 were of assistance in highlighting palisaded areas of the tumor, including the PCNA and BCL-2.

Keywords: basal cell carcinoma, double immunohistochemistry staining, proliferating cell nuclear antigen (PCNA), B-cell lymphoma 2 gene (BCL-2)

ABBREVIATIONS

H&E	Hematoxylin and eosin
IHC	immunohistochemistry
BCC	basal cell carcinoma
Ber-EP4	human epithelial antigen
BCL-2	B-cell lymphoma 2 gene
PCNA	proliferating cell nuclear antigen

INTRODUCTION

Diagnostic distinctions between BCC, basal cell carcinoma with squamous differentiation and SCC are clinically important because the risk of progressive disease is significantly higher with SCC than BCC. In addition, a trichoepithelioma misinterpreted as BCC burdens the patient with an inaccurate diagnosis that may result in inappropriate surgery [1]. Reactivity with the monoclonal antibody Ber-EP4 is capable of separating histologically similar basal cell and squamous carcinomas; expression of Bcl-2 and/or CD34 antigen is often helpful in distinguishing BCC from trichoepithelioma [1].

Case Report

A 57 year old male presented with a large mass on his left cheek, and reported some pain and two years of gradual growth. The lesional skin was punch biopsied, and analyzed utilizing hematoxylin and eosin (H&E) staining, and immunohistochemistry (IHC). After the skin biopsy results were received, a surgical excision was performed and a 15 cm length by 4.5 cm width flap repair was made.

MATERIALS AND METHODS

H&E and Immunohistochemistry (IHC)

We performed our H&E staining as previously described [4-7]. In our IHC testing, we utilized a dual endogenous peroxidase blockage, with the addition of a Dako Envision dual link (to assist in chromogen attachment). We then applied the chromogen 3,3-diaminobenzidine (DAB), and counterstained with hematoxylin.

The samples were run in a Dako Autostainer Universal Staining System. Positive and negative controls were consistently performed. Our staining was performed as previously described [2]. We performed IHC utilizing multiple monoclonal and polyclonal antibodies from Dako (Carpinteria, California, USA).

We utilized Ber-EP4; CD10, clone 56C6; CD68; cyclo-oxygenase-2(COX-2), clone CX-294; proliferating cell nuclear antigen (PCNA) and B cell lymphoma 2 gene (BCL-2), clone 124. Our vimentin antibody was obtained from Leica/Novocastra (Buffalo Grove, Illinois).

IHC Double Staining

Our IHC double stains were performed utilizing a Leica (Buffalo Grove, Illinois, USA) double staining system. Specifically, for primary staining we utilized a Bond Max platform autostainer with bond polymer refined red detection DS9390, an alkaline phosphatase linker polymer and a fast red chromogen (red staining). For our secondary staining, we utilized bond polymer refined detection DS9800, a horseradish peroxidase linker polymer and a DAB chromogen (brown staining). Positive and negative controls were consistently performed, as previously reported [2].

RESULTS

Microscopic Examination

Examination of the H&E tissue sections demonstrated a malignant neoplasm, comprised of focal aggregates of basaloid keratinocytes with hyperchromatic nuclei and minimal cytoplasm. Palisading of peripheral nuclei within the basaloid aggregates was also observed. The mitotic rate was brisk within the tumor, quantified at multiple mitotic figures per high powered (400x) microscopic field. Focal comedo necrosis was present within tumor nests. Focal squamous differentiation was also detected within the tumor [Figure 1]. The lesion contacted the lateral and deep punch biopsy specimen borders in the sections examined.

IHC Stains

Anti-human epithelial antigen (Ber-EP4) demonstrated diffusely positive, membranous and cytoplasmic staining on the basaloid tumor cells. PCNA and BCL-2 demonstrated focally positive staining, primarily in peripheral, palisaded areas of the tumor (Figure 1). Vimentin was very positive in dermal stromal areas around the tumor, and also positive in comedo necrosis tumor areas (Figure 1). Rare positive staining was noted on the tumor cells with COX-2. Focally positive staining was noted on the tumor cells for CD10. CD68 positive cells were appreciated in dermal areas surrounding the BCC (Figure 2).

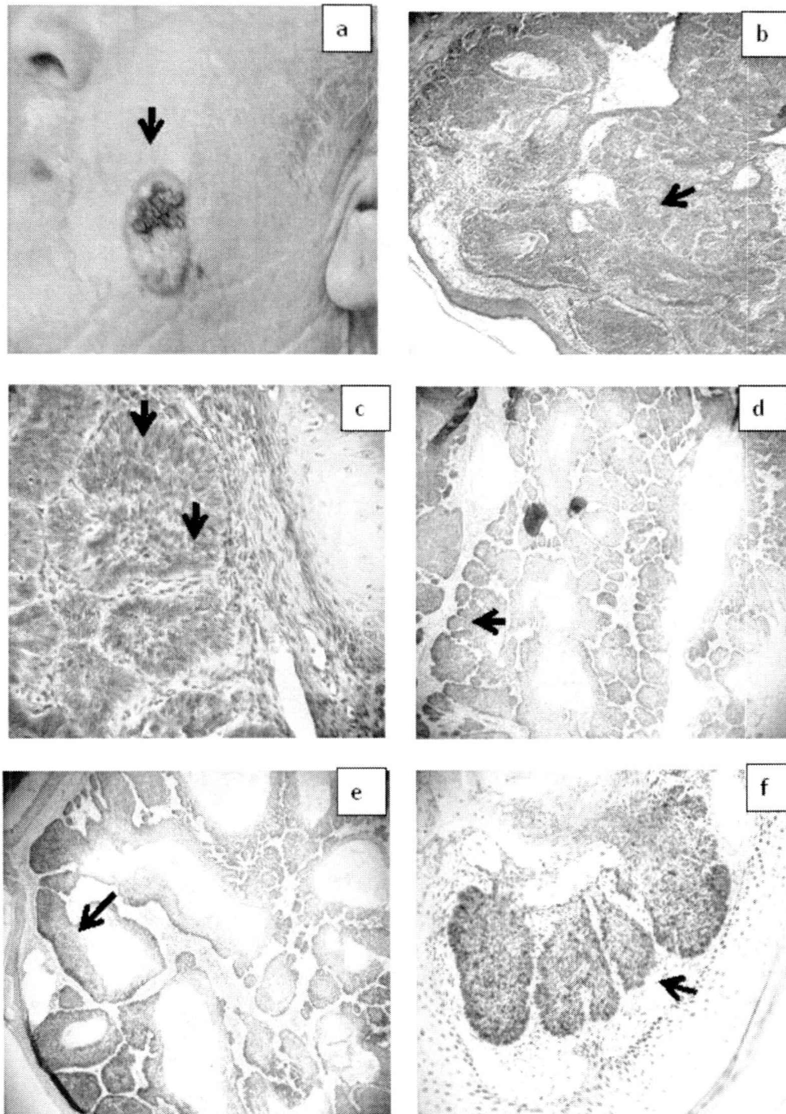

Figure 1. a. Shows the clinical BCC with central ulceration, and pearly, elevated borders (black arrow). b and c. Shows H&E stains highlighting the tumor, with palisaded peripheral tumor nest cells at 40x and 100x, respectively (black arrows). d, e and f. Show double positive IHC staining with BCL-2 in brown and PCNA in red colocalizing in the same areas (40x, 100x and 400x respectively; black arrows).

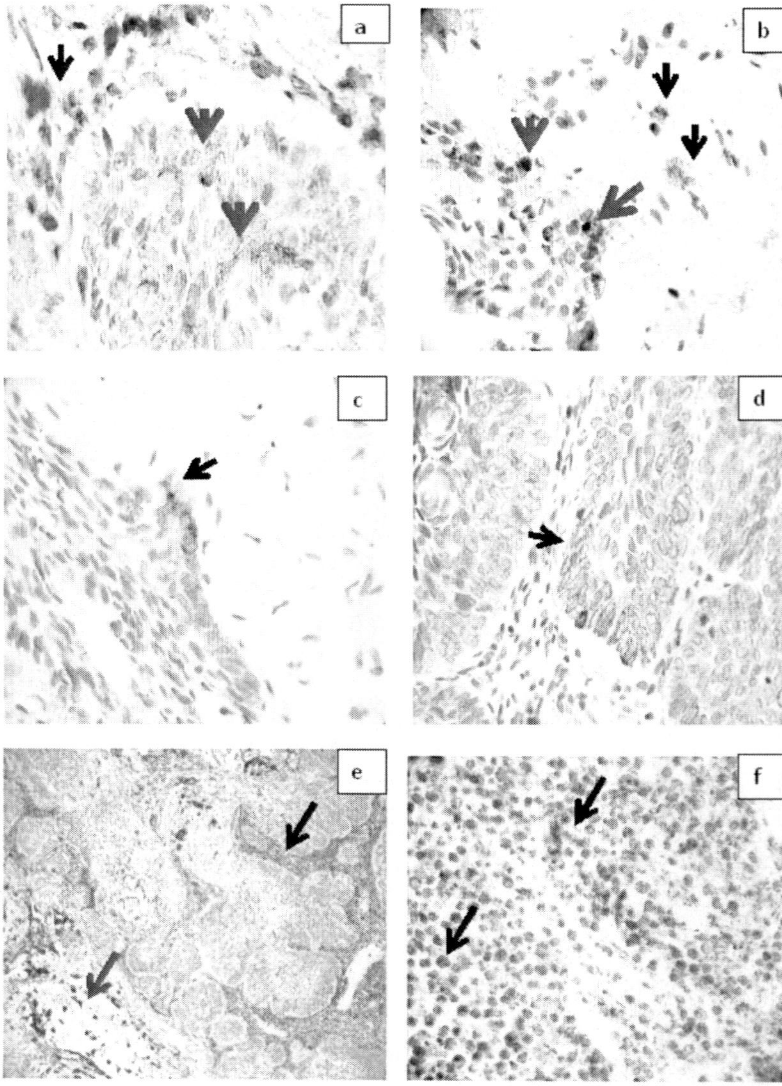

Figure 2. a. Double IHC stain with vimentin in pink (black arrow) and with CD10 in brown (brown arrows). b. Double positive IHC stain with COX-2 on tumor cells in brown (brown arrows) and a few nearby CD68 positive cells (pink staining, black arrows) (400x). c and d. Positive staining with COX-2 in brown on edge areas of the BCC (black arrows). e. Shows positive stain with vimentin in pink in the dermal peritumoral areas (black arrow) and vimentin positivity in central, comedo necrotic areas of the BCC (red arrow). f. Double IHC stain showing colocalization of vimentin in red and CD10 in brown within the tumor (black arrows).

DISCUSSION

Base on the large clinical size of this BCC, we expected to observe a brisk histologic immune response; however, we observed a mild response in an immunocompetent patient.

The monoclonal antibody Ber-EP4 is capable of separating histologically similar basal and squamous differentiated carcinomas; BCL-2 staining aids in distinguishing BCC and trichoepithelioma [1, 3-5].

One group of authors evaluated Ber-EP4, BCL-2 and PCNA stains in distinguishing BCC from SCC and trichoepithelioma [5]. In order to investigate the usefulness of these immunostains in the above differential diagnoses, the authors analyzed 45 BCCs and 22 SCCs, as well as 36 trichoepitheliomas. The authors reported that most BCCs demonstrated strong, diffuse cytoplasmic labeling with Ber-EP4, and that Ber-EP4 staining was insignificant in SCCs and trichoepitheliomas. Peripheral BCL-2 staining of trichoepitheliomas was noted in 24 of 33 of the immunoreactive tumors; the remainder marked diffusely, similar to most BCCs. The authors concluded that their data supported Ber-EP4 and BCL-2 utility in the separation of BCCs from SCCs and trichoepitheliomas. We found the proliferation marker PCNA to be positive in the palisaded areas of the BCC. The expression of proliferating cell nuclear antigen (PCNA) occurs in late G1 cells, and further increases in S-phase cells with reduced levels in G2-M cells [6, 7]. Our data indicate the active, growing nature of the peripheral, palisaded areas of the tumor.

As previously noted, the histologic immune response was minimal in this BCC. Ideally, therapeutic approaches need to be optimized to assist the immune system in infiltrating BCC tumor areas.

Conflicts of interest

None.

Funding

Georgia Dermatopathology Associates, Atlanta, Georgia, USA

REFERENCES

[1] Jimenez FJ, Burchette JL Jr, Grichnik JM, Hitchcock MG. Ber-EP4 immunoreactivity in normal skin and cutaneous neoplasms. *Mod Pathol.* 1995;8: 854-58.

[2] Abreu Velez AM, Jackson BL, Howard MS. Intraepidermal and subepidermal blistering with skin necrosis, possibly caused by etanercept in treatment of a patient with psoriasis. *Our Dermatol Online.* 2015; 6:299-03.

[3] Tellechea O, Reis JP, Domingues JC, Baptista AP. Monoclonal antibody Ber EP4 distinguishes basal-cell carcinoma from squamous-cell carcinoma of the skin. *Am J Dermatopathol.* 1993;15: 452-55.

[4] Ordóñez NG. Value of the Ber-EP4 antibody in differentiating epithelial pleural mesothelioma from adenocarcinoma. The M.D. Anderson experience and a critical review of the literature. *Am J Clin Pathol.* 1998;109: 85-89.

[5] Swanson PE, Fitzpatrick MM, Ritter JH, Glusac EJ, Wick MR. Immunohistologic differential diagnosis of basal cell carcinoma, squamous cell carcinoma, and trichoepithelioma in small cutaneous biopsy specimens. *J Cutan Pathol.* 1998;25: 153-59.

[6] Abreu Velez AM, Googe PB, Kim J, Howard MS. Markers for sebaceoma show a spectrum of cell cycle regulators, tumor suppressor genes, and oncogenes. *North Am J Med*; 2015.7: 275-80.

[7] Kurki P, Vanderlaan M, Dolbeare F, Gray J, Tan EM. Expression of proliferating cell nuclear antigen (PCNA)/cyclin during the cell cycle. *Exp Cell Res*. 1986;166: 209-19.

In: Inflammatory Markers, Oncogenes … ISBN: 978-1-63484-303-4
Editor: Ana Maria Abreu Velez

Chapter 13

Octamer Transcription Factor-2 (OCT-2) and CD25 Expression in a Recurrent Cutaneous Melanoma

Ana Maria Abreu Velez[1,*], MD, PhD., Harry D. Vildibill[2], MD, FACS and Michael S. Howard[3], MD

[1]Georgia Dermatopathology Associates, Atlanta, Georgia, US
[2]Surgical Associates of Albany, Albany, Georgia, US

Abstract

Context: Recurrent cutaneous primary cutaneous melanoma differs biologically from metastatic melanoma from noncutaneous sites into the skin.

Case report: A 59 year old female with a history of two previous malignant melanomas (MM) on her left lower leg consulted her physician for an asymptomatic, subcutaneous nodule near the sites where the previous MMs were excised.

---

* Corresponding author: Ana Maria Abreu Velez, MD, PhD, Georgia Dermatopathology Associates, 1534 North Decatur Road., NE; Suite 206; Atlanta, Georgia 30307-1000 USA; Telephone: (404) 371-0077, Toll Free: (877) 371-0027, Fax: (404) 371-1900, E-mail: abreuvelez@yahoo.com.

Materials and methods: An excisional biopsy was performed for hematoxylin and eosin (H&E) review, and for immunohistochemical (IHC) staining.

Results: Review of the H&E sections confirmed a diagnosis of an unclassified subtype, Clark level IV, Breslow thickness 4.38 mm malignant melanoma. The surgical margins were free, and no epidermal involvement was noted. IHC staining with S-100 was positive on the tumor cells; S-100 positive cells were also seen within dermal blood vessels. D2-40/podoplanin staining did not confirm definitive lymphatic space invasion. Of interest, rare tumor cells also demonstrated positive IHC staining for octamer transcription factor-2 (OCT-2). Close to these cells, inflammatory infiltrate cells positive for CD25 were also noted.

Conclusion: We speculate that the OCT-2 positive MM cells may have elicited a specific, directed immune response manifested by the CD25 positive cells. Larger studies are needed to confirm our findings.

Keywords: metastatic malignant melanoma, immunohistochemistry, Octamer Transcription factor-2 (OCT-2), CD25

Abbreviations

H&E	Hematoxylin and eosin
IHC	immunohistochemistry
DAB	3,3-diaminobenzidine
MM	Malignant melanoma
OCT-2	Octamer Transcription factor-2

Introduction

Malignant melanoma (MM) is predominantly a disease of the skin, but may present at other sites, including the mucous membranes (vulva, vagina, lip, throat, esophagus and perianal region), as well as the eye (uvea and retina) and meninges [1]. Non-cutaneous primary MMs may metastasize to the skin via blood vessels and lymphatics. The incidence of MM of the skin is increasing throughout the world, due to increased ultraviolet (UV) exposure from the sun and other UV light sources [1]. Early stage melanoma is treatable with surgery, but late stage MMs are often fatal. Metastatic melanoma usually requires surgery and cytotoxic chemotherapy as main treatment strategies;

however, these modalities are only marginally effective in the treatment of locally advanced or metastatic disease [2]. In addition to dacarbazine treatment, biochemotherapy regimens and combined chemotherapeutic agents (e.g., dacarbazine or temozolomide with vinblastine and cisplatin) and cytokine-based therapies [e.g., interleukin-2 and interferon-alpha] have been administered to induce immunogenic tumor cell death in MM patients [2]. Sentinel lymph node studies, as well as lymphoscintigraphy are also of value in the treatment of MM [3, 4].

Clinical History

A 59 year old female patient presented in June, 2015 to her surgeon with an asymptomatic subcutaneous mass on the lower left leg. The patient had a prior medical history of two (2) MMs in the same area. The patient also had a medical history of hypertension and diabetes (on both sides of her family), and was not a tobacco user. Her current medications included Effexor®, Pravacol®, Bystolic®, Neurotin®, Meloxicam®, Catapress®, and Axid.® Her mother had a history of uterine cancer. The patient had a history of a previous left lower leg primary MM, excised in March, 2013. A second left lower leg MM, likely a metastasis from the initial lesion, presented and was excised in October, 2014. In the 2014 case, a sentinel lymph node excision showed no evidence of MM.

Materials and Methods

An excisional skin biopsy for hematoxylin and eosin (H &E) review and for immunohistochemistry (IHC) stains was performed; our tissue was processed as previously described [5, 6].

Immunohistochemistry (IHC)

We performed IHC utilizing multiple monoclonal and polyclonal antibodies from Dako (Carpinteria, California, USA) as previously described [5-7]. We utilized mouse anti-human Mart-1/Melan-A/CD63, clone A103, and D2-40/podoplanin. Polyclonal anti-human S100 (reacts strongly with human S100B, and weakly or very weakly with S100A1 and S100A6, respectively) was also utilized, as well as anti-CD25 and Octamer transcription factor-2

(OCT-2) antibodies. Our CD25 and OCT-2 antibodies were obtained from Novocastra/Leica (Buffalo Grove, Illinois USA). Positive and negative controls were consistently performed.

IHC Double Staining

Our double staining was performed utilizing a Leica (Buffalo Grove, Illinois, USA) double IHC staining system. Specifically, for primary staining we utilized a Bond Max platform autostainer with bond polymer refined Red detection DS9390, an alkaline phosphatase linker polymer and fast red chromogen (red staining). For our secondary staining, we utilized bond polymer refined detection DS9800, a horseradish peroxidase linker polymer and DAB chromogen (brown staining). Positive and negative controls were consistently performed.

RESULTS

Microscopic H&E Findings

Review of the H&E sections demonstrated an MM of unclassified subtype, without epidermal involvement. The tumor presented as a single dermal mass, invasive to Clark level IV, Breslow thickness 4.38 mm, with minimal tumor infiltrating lymphocytes. No regression, tumor cell vascular invasion, or perineural invasion was noted. No tumoral ulceration, microscopic satellites, or associated nevus were identified. Neoplastic cells displayed poor maturation with progressive descent into the dermis. Individual atypical melanocytes were of small to moderate size, and displayed both spindled/fusiform and epithelioid morphologies; these cells displayed variable cytologic atypia. The atypical melanocytes contained round to oval nuclei with fine, dispersed chromatin and small, eosinophilic nucleoli [Figure 1]. Moderate amounts of eosinophilic cytoplasm were present within these cells. Frequent lesional melanocytic mitotic figures are appreciated, quantified at 1) greater than 6 per mm squared and 2) 0-5 per high powered (400x) microscopic field. The inked surgical margins were free of tumoral involvement.

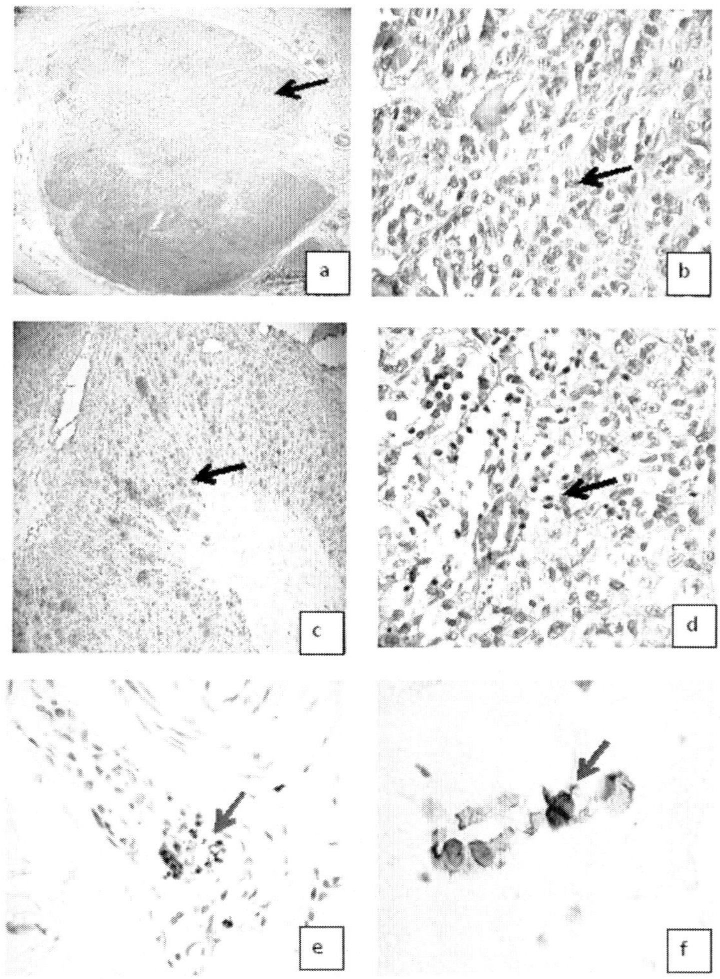

Figure 1. a and b. Shows H&E sections of the MM at 40x and 400x magnifications, respectively (black arrows). c. IHC staining, with S-100 positive staining on the tumor cells (brown staining; black arrow) (200x). d. H&E staining showing lymphohistiocytic inflammatory cells inside the tumor, in proximity to a blood vessel (black arrow) (400x). e, Positive IHC staining for S-100 inside a dermal blood vessel; the identity of these cells was not confirmed(brown staining; red arrow). f. Positive IHC staining with D2-40 on a dermal lymphatic vessel (brown staining; red arrow)(400x).

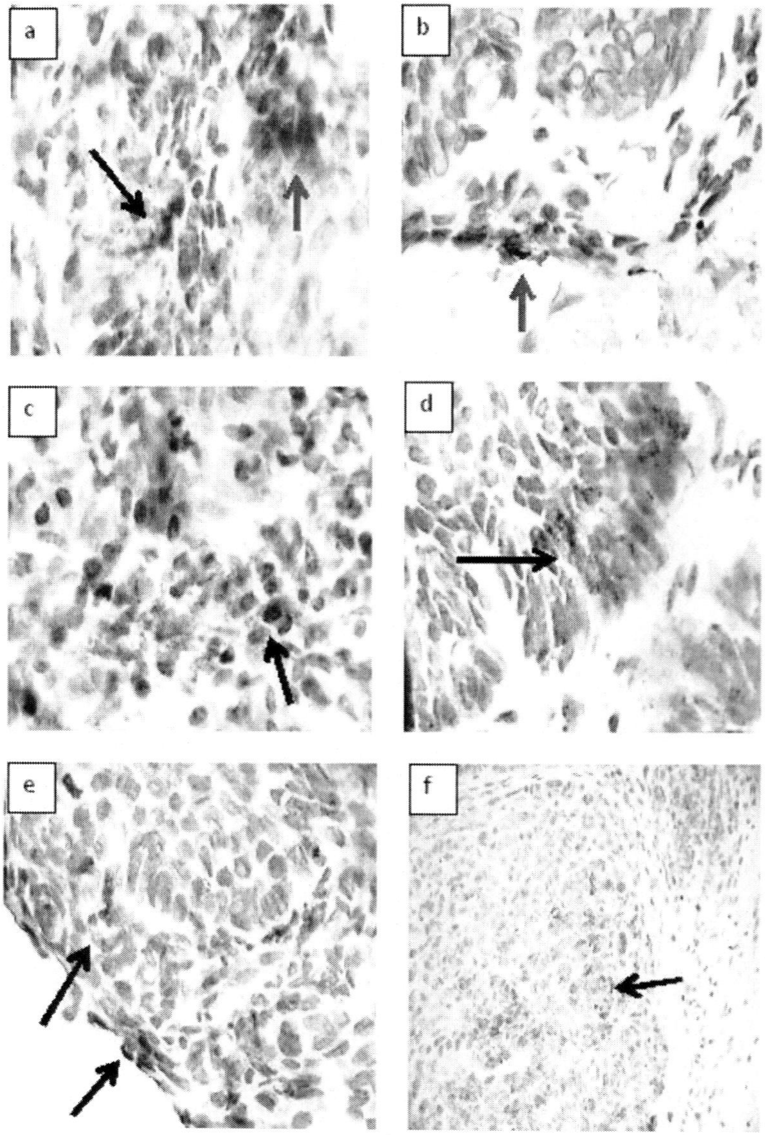

Figure 2. All IHC stains. a. Double IHC staining, showing the brown staining for Oct-2 (black arrow) and red staining for CD25 (red arrow)(400x). b. Positive staining for Oct-2 on endothelial cells next to the MM (brown staining; black arrow). c, d and e. Positive staining for CD25(black arrows). f. Positive staining for tyrosinase in the MM (brown staining; black arrow).

IHC Staining

The positive controls stain appropriately. Diffusely positive, membranous and cytoplasmic staining is noted on the tumor cells on review of the S-100 special stain. Negative staining was noted on these cells on review of the Mart-1/Melan A/CD63 special stain. No definitive angiolymphatic invasion by tumor cells was confirmed on review of the D2-40/podoplanin special stain. However, some S-100 positive cells were seen inside dermal blood vessels around the tumor (Figure 1). Sparse tumor cells were positive for OCT-2. Of interest, a few CD25 positive cells in the MM were noted in proximity to the OCT-2 positive cells (Figure 2).

DISCUSSION

In human cancer, genetic and multiple cell cycle abnormalities are complex and have been reviewed [7]. To our knowledge and having reviewed the MESH terms Oct-2, CD25 and melanoma, we present the first case of recurrent MM that it has been found to sparsely express Oct-2 in individual cells. Octamer transcription factor-2 (Oct-2) is a member of the POU (Pit-Oct-Unc) family of transcription factors, and is mainly expressed in B lymphocytes and in neuronal cells [8, 9]. POU-domain transcription factors are known as developmental regulators which control organ development and cell phenotypes [8, 9]. Other authors have noted the existence of two members of the POU domain family of transcriptional regulators, closely related to Oct-2, that are selectively expressed in terminally differentiating epidermis and hair follicles [9].

Utilizing *in vitro* MM cells, other authors have shown some expression of CD25 on some MM cells [10]. CD25 antigen, the alpha subunit of the interleukin-2 receptor, is a single-chain glycoprotein; following the activation of T cells via this receptor, interleukin-2 (IL-2) is rapidly synthesized and secreted. In addition, in response to CD25 activation, a subpopulation of T cells expresses high affinity receptors for IL-2. These cells then proliferate in an autocatalytic manner, expanding the T lymphocyte population which is capable of mediating helper, suppressor and cytotoxic functions. The IL-2 receptor is not exclusively found on T cells, and is reported to be expressed on HTLV-transformed T and B cells, EBV-transformed B cells, myeloid precursors and oligodendrocytes. Our findings may indicate a targeted immune response within a spatial colocalization where the Oct-2 expressing MM cells were present.

Further, we speculate that the CD25 positive immune cells are reacting to Oct-2 abnormal expression and trying to control dysfunctional cell regulation. Larger studies are needed to address this possibility.

ACKNOWLEDGMENT

Jonathan S. Jones, HT(ASCP) at Georgia Dermatopathology Associates provided excellent technical assistance.

Conflicts of interest

None.

Funding

Georgia Dermatopathology Associates, Atlanta, Georgia, USA.

REFERENCES

[1] Watts CG, Dieng M, Morton RL, Mann GJ, Menzies SW, Cust AE. Clinical practice guidelines *Br J Dermatol.* 2015;172:33-7.

[2] Kim T, Amaria RN, Spencer C, Reuben A, Cooper ZA, Wargo JA. Combining targeted therapy and immune checkpoint inhibitors in the treatment of metastatic melanoma. *Cancer Biol Med.* 2014;11:237-6.

[3] Intenzo CM, Truluck CA, Kushen MC, Kim SM, Berger A, Kairys JC. Lymphoscintigraphy in cutaneous melanoma *Radiographic*s. 2009;29:1125-5.

[4] Gyorki DE, Henderson MA. Sentinel lymph *Med J Aust.* 2014;201:442-4.

[5] Abreu Velez AM, Howard MS, Pereyo NY, Delman KA, Mihm MC, Rizzo M. Lymphohistiocytic CD45/CD8 immune response in a case of malignant melanoma, with possible cannibalism. *North Am J Med Sci.*

[6] Abreu Velez AM, Howard MS, Smoller BR. Antibodies to pilosebaceous units, in a new variant of pemphigus foliaceus. *Eur J Dermatol.* 2011;21:371-5.

[7] Abreu Velez AM, Howard MS. Tumor suppressor genes, cell cycle regulatory checkpoints and the skin. *North Am J Med Sci.* 2015;7:176-7.

[8] Andersen B, Schonemann MD, Flynn SE II, Singh H, Rosenfeld MG. Skn-1a and Skn-1i: two functionally distinct Oct-2-related factors expressed in epidermis. *Science.* 1993;260:78-2.

[9] Yukawa K, Yasui T, Yamamoto A, Shiku H, Kishimoto T, Kikutani H. Epoc-1: a POU-domain gene expressed in murine epidermal basal cells and thymic stromal cells. *Gene.* 1993;133:163-9.

[10] Mirjačić Martinović K, Babović N, Džodić R, Jurišić V, Matković S, Konjević G.. Favorable in vitro *J Transl Med.* 2015;13:120.

INDEX

A

B

C

D

E

I

K

L

M

N

O

P

Q

R

S

T

U

V

W

X

Y